OBSTETRICS AND GYNECOLOGY ADVANCES

ECTOPIC PREGNANCY

DIAGNOSIS, MANAGEMENT AND COMPLICATIONS

OBSTETRICS AND GYNECOLOGY ADVANCES

Additional books in this series can be found on Nova's website under the Series tab.

Additional e-books in this series can be found on Nova's website under the e-book tab.

OBSTETRICS AND GYNECOLOGY ADVANCES

ECTOPIC PREGNANCY

DIAGNOSIS, MANAGEMENT AND COMPLICATIONS

MALLORY T. CHURCH
EDITOR

New York

Library of Congress Cataloging-in-Publication Data

ISBN: 978-1-63463-260-7
Library of Congress Control Number: 2014953199

Published by Nova Science Publishers, Inc. † New York

Contents

Preface

Ectopic pregnancy is defined as gestational sac implantation outside the uterine cavity, and is estimated to account for 1.5% to 2% of all pregnancies. Although the incidence of the condition has nearly tripled in recent decades, its mortality has dropped due to early diagnosis and treatment before rupture. This book discusses the diagnosis, management and complications of an ectopic pregnancy.

Chapter 1 - The aim of this chapter is to describe non tubal ectopic pregnancies with particular emphasis on evolving strategies towards improving the diagnosis and management of these rare pregnancies. The chief concern is that these rare pregnancies are misdiagnosed and if unattended in a timely fashion they are associated with high morbidity often requiring major surgical intervention with loss of future reproductive function.

Non tubal ectopic pregnancies comprise of pregnancies at unusual locations. These ectopic pregnancies may be implanted in the cervix, cesarean section scar, cornua of the uterus, ovary or in the abdominal cavity. Ectopic pregnancies at these sites are rare. The etiology of non tubal ectopic pregnancies in most cases is unknown. Several risk factors have been described in the literature. In vitro fertilization and cesarean section constitute the major risk factors for pregnancy implantation at unusual locations. The incidence of these pregnancies is increasing world wide due to increase in assisted reproductive technology in achieving pregnancy and increasing cesarean section rate. Early diagnosis of non tubal ectopic pregnancies is difficult and it requires expertise. However, with the advances in ultrasound technology and availability of quantitative β-hCG, early diagnosis of these rare ectopic pregnancies is feasible. In the past, surgical treatment such as hysterectomy or extensive resection of the cornua was the only option. These surgical treatments were associated with significant morbidity and potential mortality and loss of reproductive function. Conservative management with preservation of reproductive function is now the preferred treatment. There is no universally agreed methodology regarding the conservative treatment of these ectopic pregnancies. All published information regarding management of non tubal ectopic pregnancies is in the form of case reports or small case series.

Different conservative or minimally invasive treatments have been attempted in the past. Medical treatment includes use of methotrexate (MTX), mifepristone, and misoprostol in termination of these pregnancies.

Other minimally invasive approaches mentioned in the literature are ultrasound guided local injection of methotrexate or potassium chloride combined with systemic MTX, dilatation and curettage, and laparoscopic or hysteroscopic excision of these pregnancies. All these conservative management modalities have been reported with high degree of success and with minimal morbidities. In all non tubal ectopic pregnancies, early diagnosis is the key as the conservative treatment in early ectopic pregnancy is highly successful and the morbidity is minimal. Conservative treatment is possible in advanced non tubal ectopic pregnancies; however, the treatment is associated with increased morbidity. Advanced pregnancies often require multiple combination treatments over a prolonged period of time with the attendant high morbidity.

Hemorrhage is one of the significant complications associated with non tubal ectopic pregnancies and it may require interventions such as tamponade with Foley's catheter in cases with cervical or cesarean section scar ectopic pregnancies. Other interventions to control acute hemorrhage in non tubal ectopic pregnancy include placement of cerclage suture in cervical ectopic pregnancy, and embolization of the uterine arteries.

These highly successful interventions to control acute hemorrhage in non tubal ectopic pregnancies have drastically reduced the need for hysterectomy.

Modern conservative treatment of these rare ectopic pregnancies has brought highly successful outcomes with minimal morbidity and preservation of reproductive function.

Chapter 2 - Ectopic pregnancy is defined as gestational sac implantation outside the uterine cavity, and is estimated to account for 1.5% to 2% of all pregnancies. Although the incidence of the condition has nearly tripled in recent decades, its mortality has dropped due to early diagnosis and treatment before rupture.

Treatment options include simple observation and monitoring, certain therapeutic drugs, and conservative or radical surgery and are currently considered to be the most appropriate and successful approach to ectopic pregnancy. The actual choice will depend on the patient's particular characteristics, symptoms and signs, and decision based on accurate and detailed information.

In earlier years, ectopic pregnancy was treated only by radical surgery, and a broad therapeutic armamentarium only became available in the late 20th century. This led directly to advances in diagnostic methods, specifically the advent of new techniques that allow uncomplicated ectopic pregnancy to be readily diagnosed with a high sensitivity and specificity. By combining the clinical analysis (risk factors; objective/subjective patient data), biological tests (human chorionic gonadotropin and progesterone dosing by radioimmunology methods), and ultrasound exams (abdominal or vaginal; Doppler study), the condition can be diagnosed early, thus preventing cataclysmic rupture of a tubal pregnancy and lessening the aggressiveness of the treatment.

Medical treatment of ectopic pregnancy is synonymous with methotrexate, although new pharmacologic strategies have been reported more recently. Gefitinib is a new drug that could play a major role in the management of ectopic pregnancy. This agent is an epidermal growth factor receptor inhibitor that has shown *in vitro* inhibition of placental cell growth. Several phase I randomized clinical trials have investigated methotrexate plus gefitinib in patients diagnosed with ectopic pregnancy, reporting that this drug combination achieves more rapid resolution and has fewer adverse reactions.

The authors provide a detailed analysis of the various therapeutic options available for ectopic tubal pregnancy. The authors will also review the indications and contraindications of this condition, but will not address ectopic pregnancies in unusual locations, as they are rare (fewer than 10%) and there is no consensus regarding the best treatment regimen.

The authors also review the literature that addresses the advantages and disadvantages of each type of treatment. Additionally, the authors will analyze the success rates, financial costs, risk of failure, prognosis of fertility with regard to the probability of subsequent intrauterine pregnancy and the risk of recurrence of ectopic pregnancy for each of the four basic approaches to treatment: expectant management, medical treatment (methotrexate and other drugs), conservative surgery, and radical surgery.

Chapter 3 - In the developed world, the rate of ectopic pregnancies has been increasing up to 2% of all pregnancies in the last thirty years. The incidence is thought to be higher in developing countries, but specific numbers are unknown.

The majority of the ectopic pregnancies involve the fallopian tube (95%), followed by ovarian site (3.2%), abdominal site (1.3%), cervical site (0.15%), and cesarean scar site. Even if in the last two decades a lot have been written about this topic, its therapeutic management still raises concerns, and, at the present moment, no guidelines exist to help choosing the best treatment.

Diagnosis: Diagnosis of ectopic pregnancy has improved significantly thanks to the advances in ultrasound technology, rapid and sensitive serum hormone assays and an increased understanding of the associated risk factors. Despite this, the diagnosis remains difficult, and an ectopic pregnancy could still be missed: this happens to 12% - 45% of them at their first admission to emergency department. That is why ectopic pregnancy remains the leading cause of death during the early trimester of pregnancy. Early diagnosis reduces the risk of tubal rupture and allows more conservative medical treatments to be employed, thus preserving subsequent fertility.

Management: Ectopic pregnancy may be managed expectantly, medically and surgically. In these days of increasing outpatient diagnosis and management it is important to remember the risks of ruptured ectopic pregnancy. Clear documentation of diagnostic and management strategies – with clinical, sonographic and biochemical assessment of the patient – is therefore important. Management is tailored to individual patients, always keeping in mind that women's preferences also depend on the way the treatment options are presented by the physician.

The activity of the ectopic pregnancy is pivotal in guiding treatment's choice. A very active ectopic pregnancy (hemodynamic failure, symptoms of rupture, high HCG) has an high risk of tubal rupture or has already ruptured and needs compulsorily a surgical treatment. For very inactive ectopic pregnancies (HCG < 1500 IU/L, plateau levels, asymptomatic woman) the best management could be a watchful wait, i.e., an intensive follow up until HCG normalization. However, in the other cases, the criteria for defining the activity of an ectopic pregnancy (i.e., pain, time of amenorrhea, hCG and progesterone level, size of hematosalpinx, and importance of hemoperitoneum, presence of a yolk sac, an embryo, or cardiac activity) and their cut off are still a matter of debate. Medical treatment is based on methotrexate, an antimetabolite, which is given at 1 mg/kg or 50 mg/m2 according to different protocols, and has a reported success rate ranging from 63% to 96.7%. Surgical treatment consists of conservative therapy or radical therapy: the first one has a 100% efficacy rate while the second one has a success rate ranging from 82.5% to 94.4%.

Subsequent fertility: Data about subsequent fertility are still to be confirmed: they all come from observational studies, conducted throughout a limited period, thus lacking adequate statistical power for definitive conclusions. Studies suggest that around 60% of women affected by an ectopic pregnancy go on to have a viable intra uterine pregnancy. The comparison between medical treatment and surgical conservative treatment did not show statistically significant differences, and the same result comes when comparing conservative and radical surgery. The risk of recurrence is 5-20%, regardless of the treatment option chosen. However, the risk is reduced after each subsequent intrauterine pregnancy.

Chapter 4 - Cervical ectopic pregnancy is a rare complication of gestation, and it accounts for less than 1 % of all ectopic pregnancies, with a reported incidence of 1 in 1000-95.000 pregnancies.

From the moment that ultrasound plays a crucial role in the diagnosis of cervical ectopic pregnancy and its differential diagnosis with abortion, the chapter pays special attention to the ultrasound diagnosis criteria.

Medical treatment of cervical ectopic pregnancy with methotrexate is well established and is widely accepted as the primary treatment. Treatment with methotrexate is effective in many cases, but in some cases pregnancy reaches 9 or more weeks. In these cases it is necessary to use other therapeutic tools to increase success rates.

The chapter also reviews the predictors of treatment failure.

Finally the chapter provides an algorithm on how to associate the different treatment options.

Chapter 5 - Ectopic pregnancy occurs when the developing blastocyst becomes implanted at a site other than the endometrial lining of the uterine cavity and the most common location is the fallopian tube.Etiology of ectopic pregnancy is unknown but risk factors includeprevious ectopic pregnancy, tubal pathology, and in-utero exposure to diethyl stilbestrol. The incidence is about 2/100 diagnosed pregnancies and ectopic pregnancy is suspected in any female of reproductive age with the early classic symptoms of abdominal pain, amenorrhea,vaginal bleeding, and unexplained syncope.Ectopic pregnancy is a gynecologic emergency and potentially life-threatening condition.Hemorrhage from ectopic pregnancy is still the leading cause of pregnancy related maternal death in the first trimester, despite improved diagnostic methods. The diagnosis is usually made clinically, based upon the imaging studies (ultrasound) and laboratory tests (hCG). The combination of transvaginal ultrasonography and serum human chorionic gonadotrophin will allow a definitive diagnosis in almost all cases at a very early stage of pregnancy, thereby permitting treatment options.The guiding principle has become a conservative approach that attempts to save the tube, rather than salpingectomy.In the absence of emergent surgical indication, medical therapy with methotrexate is an option and its overall success rate in properly selectedwomen is significantly high.

Chapter 6 - In human reproduction term pregnancy is the normal, expected outcome that culminates with the delivery of healthy descendants. The distinctive phenomenon of reproduction occurs amid a complex array of molecular, genetic, metabolic and hormonal influences contributing to successful pregnancies, although this process does not always evolves normally and highly disturbed outcomes have been reported as medical rarities since ancient times. In modern medicine, frequent accounts of rare reproductive disorders such as pregnancy loss due to Ectopic Pregnancy (EP), constitute one of the most devastating medical concerns of the last 35 years, having not only a negative impact by compromising fertility among young women but resulting also in considerable fatalities signifying great economic burden on societies world-wide. Given the alarming demographic increases of reproductive dysfunctions major ethically acceptable research efforts have been devised in humans and animal models, as they comprise an important medical tool where ongoing research has proven to be of great value to define a better understanding of complex genetic, immunologic, hormonal and metabolic factors leading to EP in women, when unknown disturbances deregulate embryotubal transport and tubal microenvironment is modified, suggesting the need to further study multifaceted risk factors of fetal loss in alternative animal models such as lagomorphs and swine, species where major discoveries have been documented. Finally, the objective of this chapter is to contribute to the current knowledge of reproductive anomalies disclosing novel related risk factors described in research in animal models, and discuss an analogous panorama of EP in the rabbit, a species that has provided well-documented rarities encompassing fetal complications and constitute a unique potential source of research resources.

In: Ectopic Pregnancy
Editor: Mallory T. Church
ISBN: 978-1-63463-260-7

Chapter 1

Non Tubal Ectopic Pregnancies - Diagnosis and Conservative Management

Usha Verma**, *M.D. and Ankita Desai, M.D.
Department of Obstetrics and Gynecology, Miller School of Medicine, University of Miami, Miami, Florida. US

Abstract

The aim of this chapter is to describe non tubal ectopic pregnancies with particular emphasis on evolving strategies towards improving the diagnosis and management of these rare pregnancies. The chief concern is that these rare pregnancies are misdiagnosed and if unattended in a timely fashion they are associated with high morbidity often requiring major surgical intervention with loss of future reproductive function.

Non tubal ectopic pregnancies comprise of pregnancies at unusual locations. These ectopic pregnancies may be implanted in the cervix, cesarean section scar, cornua of the uterus, ovary or in the abdominal cavity. Ectopic pregnancies at these sites are rare. The etiology of non tubal ectopic pregnancies in most cases is unknown. Several risk factors have been described in the literature. In vitro fertilization and cesarean section constitute the major risk factors for pregnancy implantation at unusual locations. The incidence of these pregnancies is increasing world

* Corresponding Author e mail: uverma@med.miami.edu

wide due to increase in assisted reproductive technology in achieving pregnancy and increasing cesarean section rate. Early diagnosis of non tubal ectopic pregnancies is difficult and it requires expertise. However, with the advances in ultrasound technology and availability of quantitative β-hCG, early diagnosis of these rare ectopic pregnancies is feasible. In the past, surgical treatment such as hysterectomy or extensive resection of the cornua was the only option. These surgical treatments were associated with significant morbidity and potential mortality and loss of reproductive function. Conservative management with preservation of reproductive function is now the preferred treatment. There is no universally agreed methodology regarding the conservative treatment of these ectopic pregnancies. All published information regarding management of non tubal ectopic pregnancies is in the form of case reports or small case series.

Different conservative or minimally invasive treatments have been attempted in the past. Medical treatment includes use of methotrexate (MTX), mifepristone, and misoprostol in termination of these pregnancies.

Other minimally invasive approaches mentioned in the literature are ultrasound guided local injection of methotrexate or potassium chloride combined with systemic MTX, dilatation and curettage, and laparoscopic or hysteroscopic excision of these pregnancies. All these conservative management modalities have been reported with high degree of success and with minimal morbidities. In all non tubal ectopic pregnancies, early diagnosis is the key as the conservative treatment in early ectopic pregnancy is highly successful and the morbidity is minimal. Conservative treatment is possible in advanced non tubal ectopic pregnancies; however, the treatment is associated with increased morbidity. Advanced pregnancies often require multiple combination treatments over a prolonged period of time with the attendant high morbidity.

Hemorrhage is one of the significant complications associated with non tubal ectopic pregnancies and it may require interventions such as tamponade with Foley's catheter in cases with cervical or cesarean section scar ectopic pregnancies. Other interventions to control acute hemorrhage in non tubal ectopic pregnancy include placement of cerclage suture in cervical ectopic pregnancy, and embolization of the uterine arteries.

These highly successful interventions to control acute hemorrhage in non tubal ectopic pregnancies have drastically reduced the need for hysterectomy.

Modern conservative treatment of these rare ectopic pregnancies has brought highly successful outcomes with minimal morbidity and preservation of reproductive function.

Introduction

Ectopic pregnancy is associated with high morbidity and may result in mortality if undiagnosed in timely fashion. The incidence of nontubal ectopic pregnancies appears to be rising, due to increase use of assisted reproductive technology and increase in cesarean section rate. These rare ectopic pregnancies are encountered more now and present a challenge to the treating physician. Conservative minimally invasive treatment is favored as it is associated with less morbidity and preserves reproductive function. Over the last several years the conservative treatment of tubal ectopic pregnancies has developed into a standard protocol, which is universally accepted. However, since non tubal ectopic pregnancies are rare and the information available in the literature is available only in form of case reports or small case series based on investigators experience with a certain approach, there is no well established protocol in existence.

Cervical Ectopic Pregnancy

Cervical ectopic pregnancy results from the implantation of a pregnancy in the endocervical canal. The incidence of cervical ectopic pregnancy is less than 1 % of the ectopic pregnancies [1] or between 1 in 1000 to 1 in 18,000 live births [2, 3].

The cause of cervical ectopic pregnancies remains unknown. Previous studies have shown a high incidence of prior dilation and curettage among women with cervical pregnancies [3, 4]. Recent case reports suggest an increased incidence of cervical ectopic pregnancies in women undergoing in vitro fertilization [5, 6]. In one study cervical pregnancy was found to occur in 0.1 percent of in vitro fertilization pregnancies and 3.7 percent of IVF ectopic pregnancies. [7] Other factors that may predispose to cervical pregnancy are presence of intrauterine device and uterine anomalies such as myomas or uterine synechiae.

Diagnosis and treatment of cervical ectopic pregnancy has changed dramatically in recent years. Until early 1980s, clinical diagnosis of cervical pregnancy was usually made when uncontrollable hemorrhage was encountered during curettage for presumed incomplete spontaneous abortion. Most women required emergent hysterectomy and transfusion of large volumes of blood.

Diagnosis

In recent years, the use of real-time transvaginal ultrasound examination and readily available β-hCG assays has allowed earlier diagnosis of ectopic cervical pregnancy. The incidence of cervical ectopic cases diagnosed preoperatively rose from 35% between 1978 and 1982 to 87.5% between 1991 and 1994 [8]. Early diagnosis in turn allows fertility-sparing treatment options in these cases. Women with cervical pregnancy classically present with painless first-trimester vaginal bleeding. Clinical signs of cervical pregnancy include a soft cervix that is disproportionately enlarged compared with the uterus, a partially open external os, and profuse hemorrhage on cervical manipulation. Raskin [9] suggested the following ultrasound criteria for the diagnosis of cervical ectopic pregnancy: 1)The presence of gestational sac or placental texture dominantly within the cervix, 2) no evidence of intrauterine pregnancy, 3) visualization of endometrial stripe, and 4) hourglass uterine shape with ballooned cervical canal. Timor-Tritsch et al., [10] later proposed more stringent criteria: the placenta and entire chorionic sac containing the live pregnancy must be below the internal os and the cervical canal must be dilated and barrel shaped. In 1996, Jurkovic et al. [11] proposed 2 additional diagnostic criteria to distinguish cervical ectopic pregnancy from an aborting intrauterine pregnancy residing in the cervix. First, the "sliding sign" is detected on endovaginal ultrasound examination: when the sonographer applies gentle pressure on the cervix with the probe, the gestational sac of an abortus slides against the endocervical canal. This sliding motion will not be found in an implanted cervical pregnancy. Second, peritrophoblastic blood flow from an active vascular supply to the conceptus should be demonstrated, and it requires use of color Doppler ultrasonography. The nonviable sac transiently passing through the cervix will not have peritrophoblastic flow, as it is separated from its vascular supply.

Other adjunct imaging modalities have been utilized in cases where a definitive diagnosis is difficult to make. Three-dimensional transvaginal sonography of the endometrium may enable visualization of an intact endometrium and the presence of an adjacent gestational sac located within the uterine cervix. [12] Furthermore, the utilization of MRI for confirmation of cervical ectopic pregnancies has been advocated in order to potentially better localize and characterize the pregnancy. [13] Both of these imaging modalities have been suggested to aid with diagnosis and as such two dimensional ultrasound should still be used primarily for diagnosis. Figure 1 shows a transvaginal ultrasound image of a cervical ectopic pregnancy.

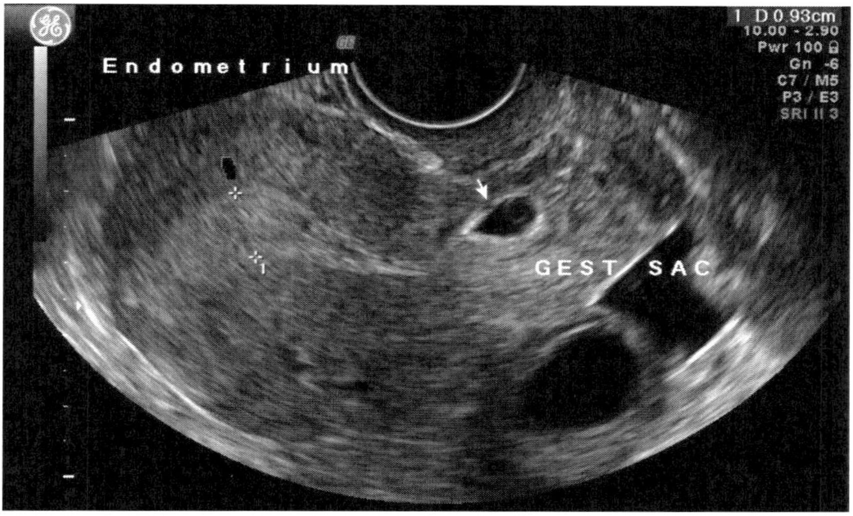

Figure 1. Transvaginal sonogram shows empty uterine cavity with a gestational sac and a yolk sac in the cervix (arrow).

Cesarean Section Scar Pregnancy

Cesarean section scar pregnancy is the implantation of pregnancy in the area of cesarean scar defect. The first case of cesarean section scar pregnancy was reported by Larsen and Solomon in 1978 [14]. The cesarean section scar pregnancy is more common than previously thought and the incidence is increasing worldwide due to increase in cesarean section rate. It constitutes 6.1% of all ectopic pregnancies and the incidence reported in the literature ranges from 1:1,800 to 1:2,216 pregnancies [15,16]. There have been two different types of cesarean section scar pregnancy proposed; one that arises from the implantation of gestational sacs on the scar with progression towards the uterine cavity and the other that manifests with deep implantation in a scar defect with progression towards myometrium and serosal layer [17]. Cesarean section scar pregnancy incidence overall is higher compared to cervical pregnancy [18]. Cesarean section scar pregnancy is believed to occur as a result of invasion of the conceptus into the myometrium through a defect in the scar. Following cesarean section, in most patients the scar is well healed and there is no defect. In some cases, however, there can be a defect in the area of the cesarean section due to poor healing and extensive fibrosis. The number of cesareans sections increases the area of scarring and defect and with multiple cesarean sections the likelihood of implantation in cesarean section scar increases. Jurkovic [15] reported that two thirds of patients with cesarean scar ectopic pregnancies had more than two previous cesarean sections. Although other authors have reported lack of association between the number of cesarean sections and the likelihood of cesarean section scar pregnancy [19, 20]. Increase in incidence of cesarean section scar pregnancy may also be due to change in surgical technique over the last several years, one layer closure during cesarean as opposed to two layer closures [20]. A single layer closure may lead to impaired postoperative healing and creation of defects within the scar [21]. Some authors have reported an association between cesarean section scar pregnancies and previous cesarean breech deliveries [17, 21-24]. The explanation suggested is that most breech deliveries are by elective cesarean section and the lower uterine segment is not well developed and that leads to impaired healing and pregnancy implantation in the cesarean section scar defect. More recently, as a result of increasing incidence, there have been reports of recurrent cesarean scar ectopic. Qian, et al., studied risk factors for recurrence in 21 women with recurrent cesarean section pregnancies in China which included a history of cesarean delivery in rural community hospitals, a thinner lower uterine segment, a gestational sac bulging into the uterovesical fold, a history of irregular vaginal bleeding or lower abdominal pain in a first-time cesarean scar pregnancy, and an early termination (≤56 days) of the first cesarean scar pregnancy. [25]

Diagnosis

The use of endovaginal ultrasound and availability of quantitative β-hCG assist in the diagnosis of these pregnancies. High index of suspicion in patients with previous cesarean deliveries and pelvic ultrasound expertise are essential to diagnose cesarean scar ectopic pregnancy. Lack of suspicion and unfamiliarity with this rare ectopic pregnancy are the most common causes for misdiagnosis. Early and accurate diagnosis is essential as late diagnosis resulting in advancement of pregnancy may result in uterine rupture. The treatment of advanced pregnancy is more complicated and is associated with increased morbidity. Patient's history and clinical manifestations of abdominal pain and bleeding may help in the diagnosis. Patient's medical history and presentation may assist in differentiating cesarean scar implantation from spontaneous abortions [16]. Most of the patients with spontaneous or inevitable abortion present with extensive bleeding and complain of cramping or lower abdominal pain while cesarean section scar pregnancy patients mostly complain of only mild or moderate lower abdominal pain and minimal vaginal bleeding. Rotas et al. [20] reported that ultrasound correctly diagnosed cesarean section scar pregnancy in 84.6% (95% confidence interval 0.763-0.905) of the cases. The remainder of the cases were incorrectly diagnosed as cervical pregnancies or incomplete abortions [20]. Vial et al. [17] suggested the following criteria for the diagnosis of cesarean section scar pregnancy: 1) The trophoblast must be located between the bladder and the anterior uterine wall; 2) No fetal parts in the uterine cavity; 3) On a sagittal uterine view that runs through the amniotic sac, no myometrium is seen between the gestational sac and the bladder, due to lack of continuity of the anterior uterine wall. Fylstra and Godin et al. [26, 27] later accepted these criteria for the ultrasound diagnosis of cervical ectopic pregnancy. Jurkovich et al. stressed the importance that there should be no healthy myometrium between the bladder and the gestational sac and use of Color Doppler imaging and negative sliding sign in differentiating cesarean section scar pregnancy from aborting conceptus. On Color Doppler imaging, the sac is well perfused in viable cesarean section scar pregnancy while aborting gestational sac will appear avascular. The negative sliding sign defined as the nondisplacement of the gestational sac from its position when gentle pressure is applied by the endovaginal probe suggests implanted pregnancy [15].

Color Doppler imaging and 3- dimensional power flow may further improve the accuracy in ultrasound diagnosis of these pregnancies by determining the flow, resistance and pulsatility indices in the trophoblast vasculature at the implantation site [28-31]. Jurkovic and his coauthors reported high velocity flow (peak velocity>20cm/s) and low impedance (pulsatility index <1) in cesarean section scar pregnancies [15]. Quantitative assessment of uterine neovascularization with 3-dimensional color imaging can be useful prior to treatment with uterine artery embolization for monitoring the response to uterine artery embolization [31]. Most of the cesarean section scar pregnancies can be accurately diagnosed with endovaginal ultrasound. Figure 2 shows a transvaginal ultrasound image of a cesarean section scar ectopic pregnancy. While previous studies have suggested that magnetic resonance imaging may have a limited role in the diagnosis of cesarean section scar pregnancy more recent studies show that there may be a role for MRI in cases in which ultrasound is limited or inconclusive [21]. In a retrospective study Huang et al. compared the detection rates with MRI vs. ultrasound. They found that the specificity of MRI in diagnosing cesarean scar pregnancy was 97.6% versus 81% of the initial ultrasound ($P < 0.05$). However, the specificity was comparable to MRI when ultrasound was repeated. [32]. As ultrasound has shown to be more readily available and cost effective it should still be used as the initial diagnostic test of choice. In undiagnosed cases, laparoscopy can be utilized in which the cesarean section scar pregnancy may appear as a bulge in the area of the cesarean section scar. Cystoscopy has been used to rule out bladder penetration [33]. Roberts et al. described cesarean section scar pregnancy as a salmon red appearing lesion [34].

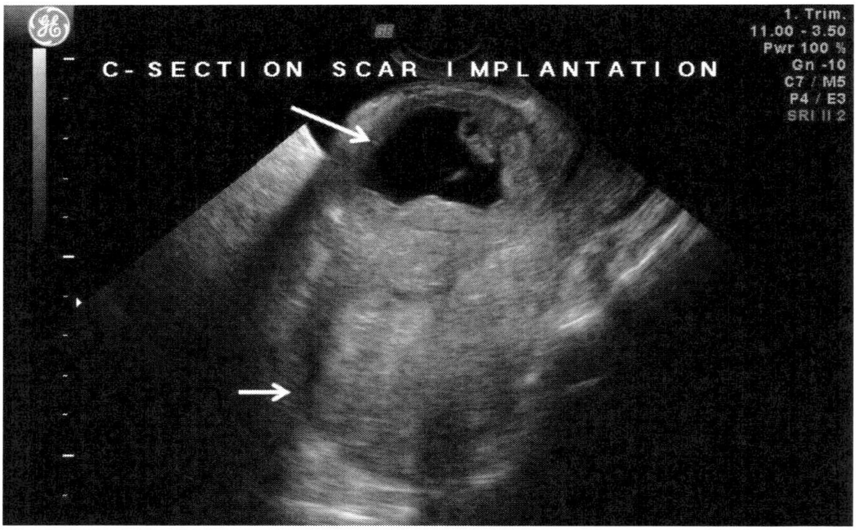

Figure 2. Transvaginal sonogram shows cesarean cesarean section scar pregnancy (larger arrow) and an empty uterine cavity (smaller arrow).

Cornual Ectopic Pregnancy

Cornual or interstitial ectopic pregnancy is an uncommon form of ectopic pregnancy. Cornual ectopic pregnancy is found in 2-4% of all ectopic pregnancies, with an estimates incidence of one in every 2500 to 5000 deliveries [35]. The predisposing factors for this abnormal location of pregnancy are rudimentary horn, previous salpingectomy, proximal intratubal adhesions, previous ectopic pregnancy, pelvic inflammatory disease, IVF, ovulation induction [36-39]. In a cornual pregnancy the pregnancy is in the area of the tubal ostia, and the pregnancy in this area can advance to second trimester before the rupture of the cornua occurs. The average size of the cornual portion of the tube is 0.7 mm in diameter and 1-2 cm in length allowing it to expand significantly before rupture [39]. Diagnosis and management at a later gestational age results in higher rates of rupture which can lead to hemorrhage and mortality, reported at 2 % in the literature which is 7 times the mortality rate of ectopic pregnancies in general [38-40].

Diagnosis

Despite the availability of transvaginal ultrasound and β-hCG assays, early identification of a cornual ectopic pregnancy remains a difficult task. Early diagnosis by ultrasound can be made by a skilled ultrasonographer. In cornual ectopic pregnancy the pregnancy is located laterally in the uterine fundus away from the classical endometrial stripe. Criteria for ultrasound diagnosis of cornual ectopic pregnancy established by Timor-Tristsch and his group are that in a cornual ectopic pregnancy the gestational sac is surrounded by a thin rim (<5mm) myometrium and the sac is an eccentric position more than 1 cm from the lateral wall of the endometrial cavity [41]. Ackerman et al. described the interstitial line sign, which has been reported to be 80% sensitive and 98% specific in diagnosing an interstitial pregnancy. The interstitial line sign is the visualization of an echogenic line that runs from the endometrial cavity to the cornual region, abutting the interstitial mass [42]. Three dimensional ultrasound imaging as well as MRI may be helpful in the diagnosis of ectopic pregnancy however further studies are needed to evaluate the sensitivity and specificities of these modalities. Figure 3 shows a transvaginal ultrasound image of a cornual ectopic pregnancy.

Ovarian Pregnancy

An ovarian pregnancy occurs when ovum is fertilized and is retained with in the ovary. Ovarian pregnancy accounts for 3% of ectopic pregnancies [43]. Risk factors include pelvic inflammatory disease, IUD use, endometriosis, and assisted reproductive technologies. The incidence of ovarian pregnancy has been reported to be higher with the use of intrauterine devices [44] Ovarian pregnancy sometimes manifests as a part of heterotopic pregnancy [45,46] and may manifest at the same time as tubal pregnancies [43]. Ovarian pregnancies can be classified as extrafollicular and intrafollicular type, of which the intrafollicular type is less common. The pathogenesis of ovarian pregnancy is undetermined. It is unknown if the pregnancy in the ovary occurs as a result of failure of follicle to rupture or due to secondary implantation of the embryo.

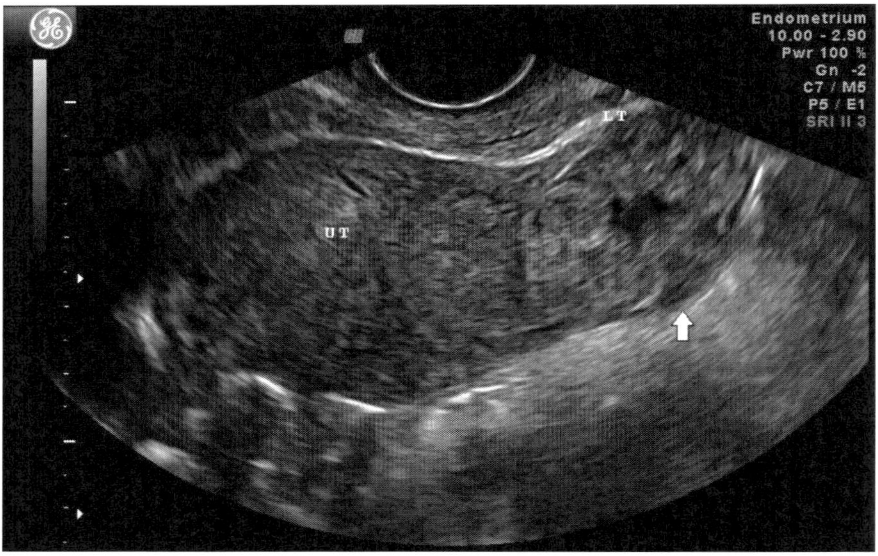

Figure 3. Transvaginal sonogram shows a left cornual ectopic pregnancy (arrow).

Diagnosis

Ultrasound diagnosis of ovarian pregnancy can be challenging. In cases of heterotopic pregnancy the ovarian pregnancy may be missed when an intrauterine pregnancy is seen on ultrasound. The features suggestive of ovarian pregnancy are presence of a gestational sac, chorionic villi, or an atypical cyst with a hyperechoic ring with in the ovary [47, 48]. Spielberg et al. proposed established criteria for diagnosis: (1) fallopian tubes including fimbria must be intact and separate from the ovary; (2) the pregnancy must occupy the normal position of the ovary; (3) the ovary must be attached to the uterus through the utero-ovarian ligament; and (4) there must be ovarian tissue attached to the pregnancy in the specimen [47]. Moreover, the addition of color Doppler is helpful, as it will show increased vascularity in the area of implantation site. The presence of a yolk sac or fetal pole in the ovarian mass will be more diagnostic. Ovarian pregnancy may be confused with corpus luteal cyst.

Three-dimensional ultrasound has been reported to be useful in differentiating ovarian pregnancy from corpus luteum cysts [49]. Ultimately however, diagnostic laparoscopy may be required to make a diagnosis of ovarian pregnancy. At the time of laparoscopy the ovarian pregnancy may resemble a hemorrhagic cyst.

Heterotopic Pregnancy

Heterotopic pregnancy occurs when an intrauterine and an extrauterine pregnancy occur simultaneously. The extrauterine pregnancy in heterotopic pregnancies is mostly tubal. Incidence of heterotopic pregnancy overall has been reported as 1/8000-1/30,000 in spontaneous pregnancies [50]. Awareness of heterotopic pregnancy is increasingly important as more women undergo assisted reproduction, particularly ovulation induction. The prevalence of heterotopic pregnancy in women who undergo assisted reproduction has been reported to be 1%–3% [51]. Its incidence is increased in women undergoing assisted conception with superovulation, IVF-ET and GIFT. [52].

Diagnosis

Heterotopic pregnancy remains a diagnostic challenge and should be kept in mind when a patient who has undergone assisted reproduction presents with pelvic pain. Ultrasound imaging can demonstrate the presence of an intrauterine and an extrauterine pregnancy. However, a retrospective study of 25 heterotopic pregnancies by Yu et al. reported that only 56% of heterotopic pregnancies were diagnosed by the initial ultrasound at 6-7 weeks [53]. As a result a high index for suspicion should be kept for patients with risk factors such as those undergoing assisted reproduction. Furthermore, if a patient undergoes an abortion of an intrauterine pregnancy and continues to experience persistent adnexal pain with abnormal β-hCG levels, heterotopic pregnancy should be suspected. The ectopic pregnancy may be in any of the locations, tubal (most common), cervical, cornual pregnancy or ovarian pregnancy. Ultimately, the diagnosis of heterotopic pregnancy may not be made until the time of surgery as shown by systematic review by Talbolt et al. in which 11% of cases were diagnosed by laparoscopy and 18% by laparotomy

[54]. High vigilance is required for diagnosis of these ectopic pregnancies in the presence of intrauterine pregnancy.

Abdominal Pregnancy

Abdominal pregnancies can be classified as primary abdominal pregnancy or secondary abdominal pregnancy. In primary pregnancy it is assumed that fertilization occurs outside the uterine adnexa. In secondary abdominal pregnancy that is presumably more common, it is believed to result from undetected rupture of a tubal pregnancy. Implantation can occur anywhere in the abdomen on any viscera even rarely implantation may occur on the liver and spleen. The incidence of abdominal pregnancy is estimated at 10.9 per 100,000 live births and 9.2 per 1,000 ectopic pregnancies in the United States [55]. It has been reported to be more common in patients who undergo assisted reproduction [56]. Maternal mortality associated with intraabdominal pregnancy is 7.7 times that of other forms of ectopic pregnancy due to significant hemorrhage [56]. Abdominal pregnancy is associated with high maternal morbidity and mortality and also high perinatal mortality. Maternal mortality reported with abdominal pregnancy ranges between 0 and 30 percent [57]. Increased mortality or morbidity in abdominal pregnancy is mainly because of the risk of massive hemorrhage from detachment of the placenta. The placenta can be attached to the uterine wall, bowel, mesentery, liver, spleen, bladder, and ligaments and the area of implantation is very vascular at these sites. The fetal outcome is poorer than the mother's with the perinatal mortality ranging between 40 and 95 percent [58]. Congenital fetal malformations are common in these pregnancies. Fetal outcome may be better with advanced pregnancy and especially if the fetus is surrounded by a normal volume of amniotic fluid [57].

Diagnosis

The diagnosis of abdominal pregnancy is complex. Early diagnosis is important for accurate diagnosis and management of this form of pregnancy with minimum morbidity.

Clinical symptoms and signs such as abdominal pain, tenderness, persistent abnormal fetal presentation and easily palpable fetal parts are more reliable in diagnosis of abdominal pregnancy than abnormally increasing human chorionic gonadotrophin since β-hCG levels may rise normally in an abdominal pregnancy [59]. Ultrasound, combined with clinical evaluation, has approximately a 50 percent success rate in the diagnosis [60]. The classic ultrasound finding in abdominal pregnancy is the absence of myometrial tissue between the bladder and pregnancy [61].

Most of the time the diagnosis is not made until laparotomy [62]. Magnetic resonance imaging (MRI) is a promising imaging diagnostic tool in diagnosis of abdominal pregnancy [63, 64]. MRI scan is helpful in providing additional information regarding the relationship between the abdominal pregnancy and the adjacent viscera. Moreover, MRI may aid in surgical planning once an abdominal pregnancy has been diagnosed [65]. Alibone et al. [60] described the following four major criteria for the ultrasound diagnosis of abdominal pregnancy: (1) demonstration of a fetus in a gestational sac outside the uterus, or the depiction of an abdominal or pelvic mass identifiable as the uterus separate from the fetus; (2) failure to see a uterine wall between the fetus and urinary bladder; (3) recognition of a close approximation of the fetus to the maternal abdominal wall; and (4) localization of the placenta outside the confines of the uterine cavity. The diagnostic errors reported in different series have ranged from 50 to 90%.

Management Options

The classic treatment in the past for non tubal ectopic pregnancies was surgical intervention which was at times drastic. This modality was associated with significant morbidity, potential mortality and resulted in loss of reproductive capability as well. More recently, attempts have been made to treat non tubal ectopic pregnancies in a more conservative manner with preservation of reproductive function in young women. Treatment options for non tubal ectopic pregnancies depend overall on the fetal gestational age, the woman's desire to maintain fertility and patient's condition at the time of presentation. Patients presenting with acute hemorrhage may require interventions to control hemorrhage in addition to the treatment needed for termination of the pregnancy. Early diagnosis of ectopic gestation is the key for controlled conservative treatment and prevention of any complications. Although conservative management is possible in advanced non tubal ectopic pregnancies, these pregnancies are associated with higher morbidity and may require use of multiple conservative modalities [66]. Conservative management of advanced non tubal ectopic pregnancy should be done at a tertiary care center with facilities available for blood transfusion and availability of emergency services for radiological interventional procedures.

Different approaches have been used in the conservative management of non tubal pregnancies. Nonsurgical treatment usually consists of a combination of medical and interventional measures.

Cervical Ectopic Pregnancies

Methotrexate, mifepristone, and misoprostol all have been used successfully to terminate and expulse the cervical ectopic gestation. Use of local or systemic methotrexate injections is most common [10, 67]. Other interventions include ultrasound-guided injection of KCL, curettage and tamponade, amputation of the cervix, cervical cerclage, Foley catheter placement in the cervical canal, internal iliac artery ligation, angiographic uterine artery embolization, intracervical carboprost injection, and needle aspiration of the products [68-73]

Methotrexate a cytotoxic antimetabolite medication has been use for medical treatment of tubal ectopic pregnancies for several years. The highly successful use of this treatment in tubal ectopic pregnancies has been extended to its use in the management of cervical, cornual and other nontubal ectopic pregnancies. Use of systemic methotrexate treatment alone is adequate for management of cervical ectopic pregnancies at early gestation [74]. Poor prognostic factors for methotrexate treatment alone include: gestational age of 9 weeks or older, serum β-hCG of 10,000 mIU/mL or higher, fetal crown rump length of 10 mm or longer, or presence of fetal cardiac activity [67]. Single or multiple doses of methotrexate can be administered depending upon the gestational age and serum β-hCG levels. In a more recent meta-analysis by Barnhart and colleagues [75] involving 26 published studies, the overall success of methotrexate was 89% in treatment of ectopic pregnancies. Multidose regimens are more successful in pregnancies with higher serum β-hCG, but are associated with more side effects [75]. Methotrexate local injection into the ectopic pregnancy combined with systemic methotrexate is expected to be more effective compared to systemic or local methotrexate alone. Mifepristone has been used in combination with Methotrexate and other interventions in the treatment of cervical ectopic pregnancies [76]. Use of mifepristone in treatment of ectopic pregnancies in combination with methotrexate has shown a higher success rate in cases with high progesterone levels and it has been shown to result in faster resolution of ectopic pregnancies in patients with high β-hCG [77, 78]. Misoprostol alone has also been reported to be successful in treatment of cervical ectopic pregnancy [79].

Alternatively, methotrexate or potassium chloride (KCL) can be injected directly into the gestational sac or fetus under ultrasound guidance. Methotrexate injection can be performed into the pregnancy along with systemic methotrexate [10, 80]. Intra-amniotic methotrexate seems to be most successful before nine weeks gestation, particularly in the absence of fetal cardiac activity [81]. The usual dose is 1.0 to 1.5 mg/kg maternal body weight. Use of intramniotic injection of methotrexate alone or in combination with intracardiac KCL injection (in patients with cardiac activity) is reported to be 100% successful in management of patients with cervical ectopic pregnancies [80]. Potassium chloride injection alone under ultrasound guidance transvaginally or transabdominally into the ectopic gestational sac or fetus has been successful in cases of nontubal ectopic pregnancies as well [82]. Nonsurgical management of cervical ectopic pregnancy using systemic methotrexate administration combined with fetal intracardiac KCL injection is an effective option in the vast majority of patients [74]. Administration of local feticide such as KCL increases the efficacy of MTX in those cases with positive fetal cardiac activity [67, 74]. Two mL (2 mEq/mL) KCL solution is injected under ultrasound guidance into the fetal heart to achieve cardiac asystole. KCL instillation under ultrasound guidance has been considered to be a safer alternative to methotrexate, especially in the cases of heterotopic pregnancies to avoid exposure of coexisting intrauterine pregnancy to methotrexate. Viable cervical ectopic pregnancies are more likely to need one or more additional procedures such as uterine artery embolization, cervical cerclage, endocervical curettage, and ligature of the uterine artery after treatment with methotrexate alone or a combination of methotrexate and potassium chloride injection [66, 83].

Angiographic embolization is mainly used to control acute hemorrhage following conservative medical management [84]. Conservative medical treatment can be combined with uterine artery embolization to decrease the risk of bleeding. After failure of medical treatment to reduce the risk of profuse blood loss, prophylactic angiographic embolization of uterine arteries can be performed before evacuation and curettage of the cervical canal [85]. Treatment of cervical ectopic pregnancies by means of bilateral uterine artery embolization and subsequent uterine curettage has been reported [86]. Uterine artery embolization combined with methotrexate treatment has been successful in the management of cervical ectopic pregnancy with vaginal bleeding as an alternative non-surgical treatment to control vaginal bleeding and preserve fertility [87, 88]

Curettage can result in massive hemorrhage; therefore, curettage should be combined with other mechanical techniques (cervical artery embolization or ligation, or balloon tamponade) to reduce the risk of hemorrhage. Curettage alone in this setting results in hysterectomy in about one fifth of patients [8, 11].

Use of a Foley catheter and tamponade is more effective in achieving hemostasis than packing [8]. In a retrospective case series of 13 patients with cervical ectopic pregnancies, Fylstra demonstrated the effective management of pregnancies ranging from 6 to 12 weeks with curettage followed by foley catheter tamponade. In his series the mean operative time was 15 minutes and none of the patients were reported to have any complications [88]. The Foley catheter should have a 30-mL balloon, which can be inflated to as much as 100 mL if necessary. Tamponade is commonly used after cervical curettage to prevent hemorrhage. There are isolated cases of conservative management of these pregnancies presenting with hemorrhage.

Conservative management by cervical cerclage was first described by Scott et al. in 1978 [89]. In the case of profuse bleeding, Shirodkar-type cervical cerclage can be performed. Prophylactic suture ligation of the cervicovaginal branches of the uterine arteries at the 3 and 9 o'clock positions of the uterine cervix prior to curettage is another option to avoid profuse hemorrhage during curettage of cervical pregnancy [90]. Conservative management is possible in advanced cervical pregnancies; these pregnancies may be associated with higher morbidity especially in the presence of placenta percreta and may require use of multiple conservative modalities [66].

Cesarean Section Scar Pregnancies

Cesarean section scar pregnancies can be managed by medical treatment such as systemic methotrexate alone, or a combination of local methotrexate injection and systemic methotrexate. The specific treatment should be determined based on the gestational age at the time of diagnosis and presence of fetal cardiac activity. Use of systemic methotrexate combined with local intracardiac KCL injection as described in the management of cervical ectopic pregnancies can be extended to the treatment of cesarean section scar pregnancies with fetal cardiac activity [74]. Doubilet et al. successfully treated cesarean section scar pregnancies with Potassium chloride injection alone under ultrasound guidance into the ectopic gestational sac or fetus. [82]. Treatment with systemic methotrexate followed by curettage has also been reported to be successful in some isolated cases [91, 92], but treatment primarily with curettage may result in severe hemorrhage requiring emergent hysterectomy or laparotomy with excision of the cesarean section scar pregnancy. Attempt should be made to control the hemorrhage by inserting Foley's catheter and tamponading the bleeding site with inflated balloon. Uterine artery embolization to reduce hemorrhage has also been described as adjunctive therapy [93, 94]

Uterine artery embolization followed by systemic or local methotrexate treatment and or curettage is another option described in the literature [92-94]. The role of uterine artery embolization is mostly in controlling hemorrhage in these pregnancies following conservative management. More recently a study by Wang et al. examined the role for surgical management of cesarean scar ectopic. They retrospectively reviewed 71 women with cesarean scar ectopic pregnancies who either underwent hysteroscopic removal of the pregnancy followed by a foley catheter for tamponade or laparoscopic removal of the pregnancy with complete repair of the cesarean scar in three layers. They reported no statistically significant different in the demographic data between the two groups and found that overall even though laparoscopy had longer operative time it offered more definitive management of the cesarean scar pregnancies [95].

Cornual Ectopic Pregnancies

Methotrexate in the form of systemic injection or local injection into the pregnancy is now the preferred treatment for the management of cornual ectopic pregnancies. In the past these pregnancies were treated by cornual resection or hysterectomy. Methotrexate treatment is safe in the management of these pregnancies. Cornual ectopic pregnancies most of the time present at later gestational age. These pregnancies are more likely to have high serum β-hCG levels and the presence of fetal cardiac activity. These later gestational age pregnancies may not respond to a single dose methotrexate treatment and may require multiple doses or a different approach, involving a combination of treatments. Some authors have suggested that interstitial pregnancies with β-hCG. levels >1000 mIU/mL should be treated with multidose methotrexate treatment [96].

Systemic methotrexate alone may not be successful in management of these pregnancies with high β-hCG. levels. Local injection of methotrexate into the sac with aspiration of the sac has been successful in resolution of these pregnancies.

Local intra-amniotic methotrexate injection in combination with multiple-dose systemic methotrexate increases the success in resolution of pregnancies with very high β-hCG levels [97]. Local injection of methotrexate results in faster resolution of serum β-hCG compared to systemic treatment [39]. The success rate with all forms of methotrexate treatment protocols is about 83% [39]. Although the most effective methotrexate protocol for conservative treatment of ectopic pregnancy is unknown. In the presence of cardiac activity systemic methotrexate administration combined with fetal intracardiac KCL injection is a viable option as utilized in the management of cervical ectopic pregnancies [74]. Potassium chloride injection alone under ultrasound guidance transvaginally or transabdominally into the ectopic gestational sac or fetus has been successful in cases of cornual ectopic pregnancies [82].

Surgical management in Cornual Pregnancies

Laparotomy is performed in cases of cornual pregnancy rupture with hemoperitoneum. This may require cornual resection or hysterectomy. There are some case reports of laparoscopic resection of cornual pregnancies. Laparoscopic resection may be assisted by direct injection of vasoconstrictive agents such as vasopressin. Some authors have described fulguration of the base of cornual pregnancy and then resecting the sac and evacuation of the pregnancy [98]. Successful treatment of cornual ectopic pregnancy by hysteroscopic resection has been described in a small number of cases [99,100]. With conservative medical or surgical management the reproductive function is preserved for future pregnancy but there is a risk of uterine rupture in these patients, more so with surgical management.

Ovarian Pregnancy

Treatment of ovarian pregnancy in the past traditionally was laparotomy with salpingo-oophorectomy or oophorectomy. Now as conservative management is favored, less invasive treatments are utilized in management of this condition. Medical management of ovarian pregnancy is possible if early diagnosed is made by ultrasound. Methotrexate has been successful in treatment of ovarian pregnancy [101]. Laparoscopic conservative treatment of ovarian pregnancy includes removal of the pregnancy and a part of the ovary [102]. Wedge resection of the ovary by laparoscopy is suggested as the treatment of choice [103].

Heterotopic Pregnancy

The treatment of heterotopic pregnancies is controversial. The aim is to allow continuation of the normal intrauterine pregnancy and termination of the ectopic pregnancy. Methotrexate treatment is obviously contraindicated in these pregnancies. Potassium chloride injection into the ectopic pregnancy under ultrasound guidance for termination of ectopic pregnancy without any effect on intrauterine pregnancy is one option [104].

If ectopic pregnancy is in the tube, laparoscopic salpingectomy can be performed without interfering with intrauterine pregnancy. Spontaneous resolution of ectopic pregnancy in heterotopic pregnancies has been reported [104].

Abdominal Pregnancy

The optimal treatment of abdominal pregnancy is not known. Patients with abdominal pregnancy usually present with abdominal pain and occasionally with acute hemorrhage. Abdominal pregnancies are usually diagnosed late either in second or third trimester and usually require laparotomy.

Treatment of abdominal pregnancy depends on several factors such as gestational age at presentation, viability of the fetus, fetal malformations, and maternal hemodynamic status. In cases of fetal demise surgical intervention is needed owing to the risk of infection and disseminated intravascular coagulation.

A delay in surgery for a period of 3 to 8 weeks after the fetal demise allows atrophy of placental vessels to occur and this may decrease the blood loss [105]. If the fetus is alive, laparotomy should be performed, regardless of gestational age or fetal condition because of the risk of spontaneous separation of the placenta and severe hemorrhage [106]. The placenta may be attached to vascular organs and the morbidity correlates with the management of the placenta. Attempt should be made to remove the placenta with effective control of the vascularity in order to reduce complications [107,108]. If the placenta is adherent to vital organs it should be left in situ and managed postoperatively with methotrexate treatment

Conclusion

Non tubal ectopic pregnancies, which were considered rare in the past, are now becoming more common due to increased use of assisted reproductive technology and increase in cesarean section rate worldwide. A high level of suspicion along with expertise in ultrasound is required to correctly diagnose these pregnancies during early stages. Most non tubal ectopic pregnancies can be managed conservatively with low morbidity. Advanced pregnancies are associated with higher morbidity and may require multiple conservative interventions or extensive surgical treatment.

References

[1] Marcovici I, Rosenzweig BA, Brill AI, Khan M, Scommegna A. Cervical pregnancy. *Obstet. Gynecol. Surv.* 1994; 49:49-55.

[2] Parente JT, Chau-su O, Levy J, Legatt E. Cervical pregnancy analysis. *Obstet. Gynecol.* 1983; 62:79-82.

[3] Shinagawa S, Nagayama M. Cervical pregnancy as a possible sequela of induced abortion. *Am. J. Obstet. Gynecol.* 1969; 105:282-4.

[4] Rothe DJ, Burnham SJ.Cervical pregnancy. *Obstet. Gynecol.* 1973; 42:675-80.

[5] Ginsburg ES, Frates MC, Rein MS, Fox JH, Horstein MD, Friedman AJ.Early diagnosis and treatment of cervical pregnancy in an in vitro fertilization program. *Fertil. Steril.* 1994; 61:966-9.

[6] Weyerman PC, Verhoeven ATM, Alberda AT. Cervical pregnancy after in vitro fertilization and embryo transfer. *Obstet. Gynecol.* 1989; 161:1145-6.

[7] Karande V.C., Flood J.T., Heard N, Veeck L, Muasher S.J. Analysis of ectopic pregnancies resulting from in-vitro fertilization and embryo transfer. *Hum. Reprod.* 1991; 6 (3): 446-449

[8] Ushakov FB, Elchalal U, Aceman PJ, Schenker JG. Cervical pregnancy: past and future. *Obstet. Gynecol. Surv*. 1996; 52:45-59.

[9] Raskin MM. Diagnosis of cervical pregnancy by ultrasound: a case report. *Am. J. Obstet. Gynecol*. 1978; 130:234-5.

[10] Timor-Tritsch IE, Monteagurdo A, Mandeville EO, et al. Successful management of viable cervical pregnancy by local injection of methotrexate guided by transvaginal ultrasonography. *Am. J. Obstet. Gynecol*. 1994; 17:737-9?

[11] Jurkovic D, Hacket E, Campbell S. Diagnosis and treatment of early cervical pregnancy. *Ultrasound Obstet. Gynecol*. 1996; 8:373-80.

[12] Sherer DM , Gorelick C, Dalloul M, Sokolovski M, Kheyman M, Kakamanu S, Abulafia O. Three-dimensional sonographic findings of a cervical pregnancy. *J. Ultrasound. Med*. 2008; 27(1):155-8.

[13] Jung SE, Byun JY, Lee JM, Choi BG, Hahn ST. Characteristic MR findings of cervical pregnancy. *J. Magn. Reson. Imaging*. 2001; 13:918–22.

[14] Larsen JV, Solomon MH. Pregnancy in a uterine scar sacculus: an unusual cause of postabortal hemorrhage. A case report. *S Afr. Med. J*. 1978; 53:142–3.

[15] Jurkovic D, Hillaby K, Woelfer B, Lawrence A, Salim R, Elson CJ. First trimester diagnosis and management of pregnancies implanted into the lower uterine segment cesarean section scar. *Ultrasound Obstet. Gynecol*. 2003; 21:220–7.

[16] Seow KM, Huang LW, Lin YH, Lin MY, Tsai YL, Hwang JL. Cesarean scar pregnancy: issues in management. *Ultrasound Obstet. Gynecol*. 2004; 23:247–53.

[17] Vial Y, Petignat P, Hohlfeld P. Pregnancy in a cesarean scar. Ultrasound *Obstet. Gynecol*. 2000; 16:592–3.

[18] Yankowitz J, Leake J, Huggins G, Gazaway P, Gates E. Cervical ectopic pregnancy: review of the literature and report of a case treated by single-dose methotrexate therapy. *Obstet. Gynecol. Surv*. 1990; 45:405–14.

[19] Chuang J, Seow KM, Cheng WC, Tsai YL, Hwang JL.Conservative treatment of ectopic pregnancy in a caesarean section scar. *BJOG* 2003; 110:869–70.

[20] Rotas MA, Haberman S, Levgur M. Cesarean Scar Ectopic Pregnancies Etiology, Diagnosis, and Management. *Obstet. Gynecol*. 2006; 107:1373-81.

[21] Maymon R, Halperin R, Mendlovic S, Schneider D, Herman A. Ectopic pregnancies in a caesarean scar: review of the medical approach to an iatrogenic complication. *Hum. Reprod.* Update 2004; 10:515–23.

[22] Hartung J, Meckies J. Management of a case of uterine scar pregnancy by transabdominal potassium chloride injection. *Ultrasound Obstet. Gynecol.* 2003; 21:94–5.

[23] Tan G, Chong YS, Biswas A. Caesarean scar pregnancy: a diagnosis to consider carefully in patients with risk factors.Ann. *Acad. Med. Singapore* 2005; 34:216–9.

[24] Neiger R, Weldon K, Means N. Intramural pregnancy in a cesarean section scar: a case report. *J. Reprod. Med.* 1998; 43:999–1001.

[25] Qian ZD, Guo QY, Huang LL. Identifying risk factors for recurrent cesarean scar pregnancy: a case-control study. *Fertil. Steril.* 2014; 102(1):129-134.

[26] Fylstra DL.Ectopic pregnancy within a cesarean scar: a review. *Obstet. Gynecol. Surv.* 2002; 57:537-43.

[27] Godin PA, Bassil S, Donnez J. An ectopic pregnancy developing in a previous caesarean section scar. *Fertil. Steril.* 1997; 67:398–400.

[28] Wang CJ, Yuen LT, Yen CF, Lee CL, Soong YK. Three-dimensional power Doppler ultrasound diagnosis and laparoscopic management of a pregancy in a previous cesarean scar. *J. Laparoendosc. Adv. Surg. Tech.* A. 2004 Dec; 14(6): 399-402.

[29] Shih J C. Cesarean scar pregnancy: diagnosis with three dimensional (3D) ultrasound and 3D power Doppler. *Ultrasound Obstet. Gynecol.* 2004; 23: 306-307

[30] Imbar T, Bloom A, Ushakov F, Yagel S. Uterine artery embolization to control hemorrhage after termination of pregnancy implanted in a cesarean section delivery scar. *J. Ultrasound Med.* 2003; 22:1111-5.

[31] Chou MM, Hwang JI, Tseng JJ, Huang YF, Ho ES. Cesarean scar pregnancy: quantitative assessment of uterine neovascularization with 3-dimensional color power Doppler imaging and successful treatment with uterine artery embolization. *Am. J. Obstet. Gynecol.* 2004 Mar; 190:866-8.

[32] Huang Q, Zhang M, Zhai RY. Comparison of gadolinium-enhanced magnetic resonance imaging with ultrasound in evaluation of cesarean scar pregnancy. *J. Obstet. Gynaecol. Res.* 2014; 40(7):1890-3.

[33] *Valley*MT, Pierce JG, Daniel TB, Kaunitz AM. Cesarean *scar pregnancy:* imaging and treatment with conservative surgery. *Obstet. Gynecol.* 1998; 91:838–40.

[34] Roberts H, Kohlenber C, Lanzarone V, Murray H. *Ectopic* pregnancy in lower segment uterine scar. *Aust. NZ* J. Obstet. Gynecol. 1998; 38: 114–6.

[35] Bonfante Ramírez E, Bolaños Ancona R, Simón Pereyra L, Juárez García L, García-Benitez CQ. Cornual pregnancy. *Ginecol. Obstet. Mex.* 1998; 66:81-3.

[36] Chopra S, Keepanasseril A, Rohilla M, Bagga R, Kalra J, Jain V. Obstetric morbidity and the diagnostic dilemma in pregnancy in rudimentary horn: retrospective analysis. *Arch. Gynecol. Obstet.* 2009; 280:907–10.

[37] Pluchino N, Ninni F, Angioni S, Carmignani A, Genazzani AR, Cela V. Spontaneous cornual pregnancy after homolateral salpingectomy for an earlier tubal pregnancy: a case report and literature review. *J. Minim. Invasive Gynecol.* 2009; 16:208–11.

[38] Tulandi T, Al-Jaroudi D. Interstitial pregnancy: results generated from The Society of Reproductive Surgeons Registry. *Obstet. Gynecol.* 2004; 103:47-50.

[39] Lau S, Tulandi T. Conservative medical and surgical management of interstitial ectopic pregnancy. *Fertil. Steril.* 1999; 72:207-15.

[40] Rock J, Thompson J. Telinde's Operative Gynecology. 9th ed. Philadelphia, PA: Lippincott-Raven; 2003.

[41] Timor-TritschIE, Monteagudo A, Matera C, Veit CR. Sonographic evolution of cornual pregnancies treated without surgery. *Obstet. Gynecol.* 1992; 79:1044–9.

[42] Ackerman T.E., Levi C.S., Dashefsky S.M., Holt S.C., Lindsay D.J. Interstitial line: sonographic finding in interstitial (cornual) ectopic pregnancy. *Radiology* 1993; 189(1): 83–87.

[43] Bouyer J, Coste J, Fernandez H, Pouly JL, Job-Spira N. Sites of ectopic pregnancy: a 10 year population-based study of 1800 cases. *Hum. Reprod.* 2002; 17:3224–30.

[44] Herbertsson G, Magnusson SS, Benediktsdottir K. Ovarian pregnancy and IUCD use in a defined complete population. *Acta. Obstet. Gynecol. Scand*1987; 66:607–10.

[45] Hirose M, Nomura T, Wakuda K, Ishiguro T, Yoshida Y. Combined intrauterine and ovarian pregnancy: a case report. A*sia Oceania J. Obstet. Gynaecol.* 1994; 20:25–9.

[46] Melilli GA, Avantario C, Farnelli C, Papeo R, Savona A.Combined intrauterine and ovarian pregnancy after in vitro fertilization and embryo transfer: a case report. *Clin. Exp. Obstet. Gynecol.* 2001; 28:100–1.

[47] Spiegelberg O. Zur casuistic der ovarialschwangerschaft. *Arch. Gynaekol.* 1878; 13: 73.

[48] Sergent F, Mauger-Tinlot F, Gravier A, Verspyck E, Marpeau L. Ovarian pregnancies: reevaluation of diagnostic criteria [in French]. *J. Gynecol. Obstet. Biol. Reprod.* (Paris) 2002; 31:741–6.

[49] Ghi T, Banfi A, Marconi R et al. Three-dimensional sonographic diagnosis of ovarian pregnancy. *Ultrasound Obstet. Gynecol* 2005; 26:102-4.

[50] Ceci O, Caradonna F, Loizzi P, Lobascio A, Bratta FG, Ferreri R, et al. Ultrasound diagnosis of heterotopic pregnancy with viable fetuses. Eur. *J. Obstet. Gynecol. Reprod. Biol.*1993; 52:229–31.

[51] Fernandez H, Gervaise A. Ectopic pregnancy after infertility treatment: modern diagnosis and therapeutic strategy. *Hum. Reprod. Update*2004; 10:503–13.

[52] Ojeme Selo DO, GoodFellow CF. Simultaneous intrauterine and ovarian pregnancy following treatment with clomiphene citrate. *Arch. Gynecol. Obstet.* 2002; 266:232–4.

[53] Yu Y, Xu W, Xie Z, Huant Q, Li S. Management and outcome of 25 heterotopic pregnancies in Zhejiang, China. Eur J Obstet Gynecol Reprod Biol 2014; pii: S0301-2115(14)00277-2. doi: 10.1016/j.ejogrb.2014.04.046

[54] Talbot K, Simpson R, Price N, Jackson SR. Heterotopic pregnancy. *J. Obstet. Gynaecol.* 2011; 31(1): 7-12.

[55] Atrash HK, Friede A, Hogue CJ. Abdominal pregnancy in the United States: frequency and maternal mortality. *Obstet. Gynecol.* 1987; 69:333–7.

[56] Rojansky N, Schenker JG. Heterotopic pregnancy and assisted reproduction: an update. *J. Assist. Reprod. Genet.* 1996; 13:594–601.

[57] Martin JN, McCaul JF. Emergent management of abdominal pregnancy. *Clin. Obstet. Gynecol.* 1990; 33:438–47.

[58] Ang LP, Tan AC, Yeo SH. Abdominal pregnancy: A case report and literature review. *Singapore Med. J.* 2000; 41:454–7.

[59] Costa SD, Presley J, Bastert G. Advanced abdominal pregnancy. *Obstet. Gynecol. Surv.* 1991; 46:515–25.

[60] Allibone GW, Fagan CJ, Porter SC. The sonographic features of intra-abdominal pregnancy. *J. Clin. Ultrasound.* 1981; 9:383–7.

[61] Varma R, Mascarenhas R, Jame D. Successful outcome of advanced abdominal pregnancy with exclusive omental insertion. *Ultrasound Obstet. Gynecol.* 2003; 21:192-4.

[62] Onan M A. Turp A B. Saltik A, Akyurek N, Taskiran C, Himmetoglu O. Primary omental pregnancy: case report. *Hum. Reprod.* 2005; 20:807-9.
[63] Jazayeri A, Davis T A. Contreras D N. Diagnosis and management of abdominal pregnancy. a case report. *J. Reprod. Med.* 2002; 47:1047-9.
[64] Rahaman J, Berkowitz R, Mitty H, Gaddipati S, Brown B, Nezhat F. Minimally invasive management of an advanced abdominal pregnancy. *Obstet. Gynecol.* 2004; 103: 1064-8.
[65] Köroğlu M, Kayhan A, Soylu FN, Erol B, Schmid-Tannwald C, Gürses C, Karademir İ, Ernst R, Yousuf A, Oto A. MR imaging of ectopic pregnancy with an emphasis on unusual implantation sites. *Jpn. J. Radiol.* 2013; 31(2): 75-80.
[66] Verma U and Maggiorotto F.Conservative management of second-trimester cervical ectopic pregnancy with placenta percreta. *Fertil. Steril.* 2007; 697:pp. e13–e16.
[67] Hung TH, Jeng CJ, Yang YC, Wang KG and Lan CC. Lan.Treatment of cervical pregnancy with methotrexate. Int. *J. Obstet. Gynecol.* 1996; 53:243–7.
[68] Monteagudo A, Minior VK, Stephenson C, Monda S and Timor-Tritsch IE. Non-surgical management of live ectopic pregnancy with ultrasound-guided local injection: a case series. *Ultrasound Obstet. Gynecol.* 2005; 25:282–8.
[69] Garaham D and Quaye M. Interventional ultrasound in gynecology. In: J.A. Rock and J.D. Thompson, Editors, Te Linde's operative gynecology (8th ed.), Lipponcott Raven, Philadelphia 1997:115–26.
[70] Yitzhak M, Orvieto R, Nitke S, Neuman-Levin M, Ben-Rafael Z and Schoenfeld, A. Case report: cervical pregnancy-a conservative stepwise approach. *Hum. Reprod.* 1999; 14:847–9.
[71] Chen D, Kligman I, Rosenwaks Z. Heterotopic cervical pregnancy successfully treated with transvaginal ultrasound guided aspiration and cervical stay sutures. *Fertil. Steril.* 2001; 75:1030–3.
[72] Nappi C, D'Elia A, Di Carlo C, Giordano E, De Placido G. Conservative treatment by angiographic uterine artery embolization of a 12-week cervical ectopic pregnancy. *Hum. Reprod.* 1999; 14:1118–21.
[73] De La Vega GA, Avery C, Nemiroff R, Marchiano D. Treatment of early cervical pregnancy with cerclage, carboprost, curettage, and balloon tamponade. *Obstet. Gynecol.* 2007; 109:505–7.
[74] Verma U, Goharkhay N. Conservative management of cervical ectopic pregnancy *Fertil. Steril* .2009; 91:671-4.

[75] Barnhart K, Gosman G, Ashby R, Sammel M. The medical management of ectopic pregnancy: A meta-analysis comparing "single dose" and "multidose" regimens. *Obstet. Gynecol.* 2003; 101:778.

[76] Bakour SH, Thompson PK, Khan KS. Successful conservative management of cervical ectopic pregnancy with combination of methotrexate, mifepristone, surgical evacuation and tamponade using a double balloon three-way catheter. *J. Obstet. Gynaecol.* 2005; 25: 616-8.

[77] Rozenberg P, Chevret S, Camus E, de Tayrac R, Garbin O, de Poncheville L, et al. Medical treatment of ectopic pregnancies: a randomized clinical trial comparing methotrexate-mifepristone and methotrexate-placebo. *Hum. Reprod.* 2003; 18:1802–8.

[78] Gazvani MR, Baruah DN, Alfirevic Z, Emery SJ. Mifepristone in combination with methotrexate for the medical treatment of tubal pregnancy: a randomized, controlled trial. *Hum. Reprod.* 1998; 13:1987–90.

[79] C.Gurkan Zorlu, Mehmet Simsek. Successful termination of a cervical pregnancy with misoprostol. Eur j obs gynecol Inanc Mendilcioglu. Volume 106, Issue 1, Page 96 (10 January 2003).

[80] Jeng CJ, KO ML, Shen J, Transvaginal ultrasound- guided treatment of cervical pregnancy. *Obstet. Gynecol.* 2007; 109:1076-82.

[81] Mantelenakis S, Tsalikis T, Grimbizis G, et al. Successful pregnancy after treatment of cervical pregnancy with methotrexate and curettage. *J. Reprod. Med.* 1995; 40:409-14.

[82] Doubilet PM, Benson CB, Frates MC, Ginsburg E. Sonographically guided minimally invasive treatment of unusual ectopic pregnancies. *J. Ultrasound Med.* 2004; 23:359-70.

[83] Kung FT, Chang SY. Efficacy of methotrexate treatment in viable and nonviable cervical pregnancies *American Journal of Obstetrics & Gynecology* 1999:181; 1438-44.

[84] Frates MC, Benson CB, Doubilet PM, Di Salvo DN, Brown DL, Laing FC. Cervical ectopic pregnancy: results of conservative treatment. *Radiology*.1994; 191:773-5.

[85] C.Nappi, A. d'Elia, C. Di Carlo, E. Giordano, G. De Placido and V. Iaccarino, Conservative treatment by angiographic uterine artery embolization of 12 week cervical ecotpic pregnancy. *Hum. Reprod.* 1999; 14:1118–21.

[86] Martinell P, Maroutti GM, Opppesdiano R, Agangi A, Mazzarelli LL, Votino C, Quarantelli M, Iaccarino V. Is uterine artery embolization for

cervical ectopic pregnancy always safe? *Journal of Minimally Invasive Gynecology* 2007; 14:758-63.

[87] Hirakawa M, Tajima T, Yoshimitsu K, Irie H, Ishigami K, Yahata H, Wake N, Honda H. Uterine artery embolization along with the administration of methotrexate for cervical ectopic pregnancy: technical and clinical outcomes. *Am.* 2009; 192:1601-7.

[88] Fylstra DL. Cervical pregnancy: 13 cases treated with suction curettage and balloon tamponade. *Am. J. Obstet. Gynecol.* 2014; 210:581.e1-5.

[89] Scott J, Diggory P, Edelman P. Management of cervical pregnancy with circumsuture and intracervical obturator, *BMJ.* 1978: 1:825.

[90] Saygili Yilmaz ES, Aydin D, Ylmaz Z. Conservative treatment of cervical pregnancy by evacuation after transvaginal suture ligation of cervicovaginal branches of uterine arteries, *Acta. Obstet. Gynecol. Scand* 2002; 81:988–90.

[91] Graesslin O, Dedecker F, Quereux C, Gabriel R. Conservative treatment of ectopic pregnancy in a cesarean scar. *Obstet. Gynecol.* 2005; 105: 869-71.

[92] Marchiole P, Gorlero F, De Caro G. Intramural pregnancy embedded in a previous cesarean section scar treated conservatively. *Ultrasound Obstet. Gynecol.* 2004; 23: 305-9.

[93] Yang M-J, Jeng M-H. Combination of transarterial embolisation of uterine arteries and conservative surgical treatment for pregnancy in a cesarean section scar. A report of 3 cases. *J. Reprod. Med.* 2003; 48:213-6.

[94] Sugawara J, Senoo M, Chisaka H, Yaegashi N, Okamura K. Successful Conservative Treatment of a Cesarean Scar Pregnancy with uterine artery embolization. *Tohoku J. Exp. Med.* 2005; 206:261-5.

[95] Wang G, Liu X, Bi F, Yin L, Sa R, Wang D, Yang Q. Evaluation of the efficacy of laparoscopic resection for the management of exogenous cesarean scar pregnancy. *Fertility and Sterility* 2014; 101:1501-1507

[96] Barnhart K, Spandorfer S, Coutifaris C. Medical treatment of interstitial pregnancy. A report of three unsuccessful cases. *J. Reprod. Med.* 1997; 42:521-4.

[97] Fisch J D. Ortiz B, Tazuke S, Chitkara U, Giudice L.Medical management of interstitial ectopic pregnancy: a case report and literature review. *Hum. Reprod.* 1998; 13: 1981-6.

[98] Walid MS, Heaton RL.Diagnosis and laparoscopic treatment of cornual ectopic pregnancy. *Ger. Med. Sci.* 2010; 8:Doc16.

[99] Meyer W R. Mitchell D. Hysteroscopic removal of an interstitial ectopic gestation. A case report. *J. Reprod. Med.* 1989; 34:928-9.

[100] Zhang X, Xinchang L, Fan H. Interstitial pregnancy and transcervical curettage. *Obstet. Gynecol.* 2004; 104:1193-5.

[101] Habbu J, Read MD."Ovarian pregnancy successfully treated with methotrexate.". *J. Obstet. Gynaecol.* 2006; 6:587-8.

[102] Odejinmi F, Rizzuto MI, Macrae R, Olowu O, Hussain M.."Diagnosis and laparoscopic management of 12 consecutive cases of ovarian pregnancy and review of literature." .*J. Minim. Invasive Gynecol.* 2009; 16:354-9.

[103] Raziel A, Schachter M, Mordechai E, Friedler S, Panski M, Ron-El R.. "Ovarian pregnancy-a 12-year experience of 19 cases in one institution.".*Eur. J. Obstet. Gynecol. Reprod. Biol.* 2004; 114:92-6.

[104] Fernandez H, Lelaidier C, Doumerc S, Fournet P, Olivennes F, Frydman R. Nonsurgical treatment of heterotopic pregnancy: a report of six cases. *Fertil. Steril.1993*; 60: 428-32.

[105] Meinert J. Advanced ectopic pregnancy including combined ectopic and intrauterine pregnancy [in German] *Geburtshilfe Frauenheikd.*1981; 41:490–5.

[106] Maas DA, Slabber CF. Diagnosis and treatment of advanced extra-uterine pregnancy. *S Afr. Med. J.* 1975; 49:2007–10.

[107] Varma R, Mascarenhas R, Jame D. Successful outcome of advanced abdominal pregnancy with exclusive omental insertion. *Ultrasound Obstet. Gynecol.* 2003; 21:192-4.

[108] Rahman M S. Al-Suleiman S, Rahman J, Al-Sibai M H. Advanced abdominal pregnancy-observations in 10 cases. *Obstet. Gynecol.* 1982; 59:366-72.

In: Ectopic Pregnancy
Editor: Mallory T. Church
ISBN: 978-1-63463-260-7

Chapter 2

Therapeutic Alternatives in Ectopic Tubal Pregnancy

María Teresa Gómez García*[*1], Jessica Nogueira García[2], Esther López Del Cerro[3], Ana María Castillo Cañadas[4], Esther Ruiz Sánchez[5], Carolina Serrano Diana[6] and Gaspar González Merlo[7]

[1]Obstetrics and Gynecology Department of the University and Hospital Complex of Albacete, Spain
Medical Science Department, School of Medicine of Albacete, Universidad de Castilla-La Mancha, Spain
[2,3]Obstetrics and Gynecology Department, Hospital La Plana of Villarreal (Castellón), Spain
[4,5,6] Obstetrics and Gynecology Department, University and Hospital Complex of Albacete, Spain
[7]Obstetrics and Gynecology Department of the University and Hospital Complex of Albacete, Spain and
Medical Science Department, School of Medicine of Albacete, Universidad de Castilla-La Mancha, Spain

[*] tgomezg67@gmail.com

Abstract

Ectopic pregnancy is defined as gestational sac implantation outside the uterine cavity, and is estimated to account for 1.5% to 2% of all pregnancies. Although the incidence of the condition has nearly tripled in recent decades, its mortality has dropped due to early diagnosis and treatment before rupture.

Treatment options include simple observation and monitoring, certain therapeutic drugs, and conservative or radical surgery and are currently considered to be the most appropriate and successful approach to ectopic pregnancy. The actual choice will depend on the patient's particular characteristics, symptoms and signs, and decision based on accurate and detailed information.

In earlier years, ectopic pregnancy was treated only by radical surgery, and a broad therapeutic armamentarium only became available in the late 20th century. This led directly to advances in diagnostic methods, specifically the advent of new techniques that allow uncomplicated ectopic pregnancy to be readily diagnosed with a high sensitivity and specificity. By combining the clinical analysis (risk factors; objective/subjective patient data), biological tests (human chorionic gonadotropin and progesterone dosing by radioimmunology methods), and ultrasound exams (abdominal or vaginal; Doppler study), the condition can be diagnosed early, thus preventing cataclysmic rupture of a tubal pregnancy and lessening the aggressiveness of the treatment.

Medical treatment of ectopic pregnancy is synonymous with methotrexate, although new pharmacologic strategies have been reported more recently. Gefitinib is a new drug that could play a major role in the management of ectopic pregnancy. This agent is an epidermal growth factor receptor inhibitor that has shown *in vitro* inhibition of placental cell growth. Several phase I randomized clinical trials have investigated methotrexate plus gefitinib in patients diagnosed with ectopic pregnancy, reporting that this drug combination achieves more rapid resolution and has fewer adverse reactions.

We provide a detailed analysis of the various therapeutic options available for ectopic tubal pregnancy. We will also review the indications and contraindications of this condition, but will not address ectopic pregnancies in unusual locations, as they are rare (fewer than 10%) and there is no consensus regarding the best treatment regimen.

We also review the literature that addresses the advantages and disadvantages of each type of treatment. Additionally, we will analyze the success rates, financial costs, risk of failure, prognosis of fertility with regard to the probability of subsequent intrauterine pregnancy and the risk of recurrence of ectopic pregnancy for each of the four basic approaches to treatment: expectant management, medical treatment (methotrexate and other drugs), conservative surgery, and radical surgery.

Introduction

Ectopic pregnancy is defined as gestational sac implantation outside the uterine cavity, and is estimated to account for 1.5% to 2% of all pregnancies [1]. Tubal ectopic pregnancy is the most common of all blastocyst implantation disorders: at least 90% of all ectopic pregnancies occur in the fallopian tube, and 80% implant in the ampullary portion of the fallopian tube [2]. The condition has become more common in recent decades, mainly due to assisted-reproduction techniques, although this rise has fortunately not been accompanied by higher rates of mortality or severe morbidity. Early diagnosis before fallopian tube rupture and greater treatment efficacy have lowered mortality [1], although tubal ectopic pregnancy still accounts for 4% of maternal deaths in the U.S. in the early 21st century [3].

The current therapeutic armamentarium includes expectant management of tubal ectopic pregnancy, medical treatment with methotrexate (MTX) at different doses and via different routes of administration, conservative surgery (salpingostomy), radical surgery (salpingectomy), and new medical strategies (mifepristone, gefitinib). In 2014, treatment innovations are related to the choice of one or another therapeutic option. A new concept called “ectopic pregnancy activity” has recently been defined, but is still a topic of debate. Nevertheless, this concept will apparently become a decisive factor when choosing the most appropriate and most beneficial treatment for the patient [4].

Capmas et al. [4] considered the activity level of ectopic pregnancy to be the main factor when deciding on treatment. These authors differentiate between “active ectopic pregnancy”, “less active ectopic pregnancy” and “very less active ectopic pregnancies”. Active ectopic pregnancy is characterized by a high risk of fallopian tube rupture or by actual rupture. It also includes hemodynamically unstable patients with symptoms of rupture (pain or syncope) or high β-hCG levels (although “high” has not yet been defined). There is consensus on this kind of patient, and it is generally agreed that surgery is the most appropriate treatment in these cases.

The same authors propose defining less active ectopic pregnancy as patients who are hemodynamically stable and have mild or no symptoms, pretreatment serum β-hCG levels < 5000 IU/L, and no embryonic cardiac activity. As a whole, this group of ectopic pregnancy is eligible for medical treatment. Lastly, the group of very less active ectopic pregnancies could be defined as those with low serum β-hCG levels (< 1500 IU/L) that are dropping or have plateaued. This group would also include pregnancies of unknown location that meet the same criteria for β-hCG levels. In principle, these inactive ectopic pregnancies would benefit from expectant management.

We review the indications for each of the different therapeutic options and present the success rates, economic costs, risk of failure, prognosis of fertility in terms of probability of subsequent intrauterine pregnancy, risk of another ectopic pregnancy, patient preferences (new variable not previously considered), and follow-up time to full cure.

Expectant Management

In 1884, Lawson Tait [5] presented the first series of ectopic pregnancies (5 cases) treated by surgery immediately before or at the time of fallopian tube rupture. In his first patient, Tait confirmed a ruptured left tubal ectopic pregnancy, but the bleeding was uncontrollable and led to intraoperative death. However, the other four patients underwent salpingectomy and progressed satisfactorily. Tait was the first surgeon to treat his patients by surgery. Until then, ectopic pregnancy had never been treated but was not always fatal, and some patients experienced spontaneous resolution due to regression or tubal abortion. This scientific evidence lent support to the hypothesis that some patients could benefit from avoiding therapy and the inherent risks of surgery, anesthetic complications, and adverse drug reactions. This literature review will provide up-to-date information and identify the profile of the ideal candidate most likely to have a successful outcome when therapy is not used.

The first author to report his experience in this field was Lund [6] in 1955. The investigator selected 119 patients with a positive pregnancy test and a clinical diagnosis of ectopic pregnancy who were hemodynamically stable and had few symptoms. During a rather lengthy hospital stay, patients were monitored exclusively by complete blood count, pregnancy test, and serial physical examinations. The results were not encouraging: 57% (68 cases) of patients progressed satisfactorily and experienced spontaneous regression but the remaining 43% required emergency or acute-care surgery based on their clinical course. Although the Lund study observed high failure rates and used less-than-rigorous criteria for patient diagnosis and inclusion, this early paper opened up the field of research in the expectant management of ectopic pregnancy.

The next study was published by Mashiach et al. [7] in 1982 and included a limited number of patients (5 cases; 4 of them successfully resolved with expectant management). However, all the ectopic pregnancies were diagnosed by laparoscopy and serial serum β-hCG determinations, which led to the use of the latter as a crucial factor for patient inclusion in this type of therapeutic trial.

Since then, the literature has seen a plethora of reports on patients diagnosed with ectopic pregnancy and managed expectantly. Lund [6] first described this in 1955, and by 2004, 17 papers had been published and are summarized in Craig and Khan [8]. A total of 700 patients were included, with a success rate of 69% (range, 47%-100%). The main issue was the vast differences in the studies, which had no clear inclusion criteria, used a variety of diagnostic and follow-up methods, and observed highly variable outcomes.

Among all the articles published by 2004, only two well-designed studies compared expectant management with medical treatment. One was a double-blind clinical trial conducted by Korhonen et al. [9] to compare expectant management with low-dose MTX. This study included 60 patients diagnosed with ectopic pregnancy by vaginal ultrasound and serum β-hCG levels. The inclusion criteria were as follows: a) mild symptoms, b) β-hCG increase < 50% in 48 hours, c) ectopic pregnancy diameter < 40 mm, d) no ultrasound signs of intra-abdominal bleeding, and e) no other reason for laparoscopy. Patients were randomized to oral MTX 2.5 mg for 5 days or oral placebo for 5 days. Patients were then monitored by serial tests every 48 hours (complete blood count, chemistry, β-hCG levels) and vaginal ultrasound at 5 and 12 days. Surgical laparoscopy was performed in cases of abdominal pain and/or intra-abdominal hemorrhaging diagnosed by ultrasound. Laparoscopy was not required for cure in 77% of patients in each group. There were no differences in recovery time between the groups. Mean serum β-hCG levels were low at 211 IU/L (range, 20-1343) in the group managed expectantly and 395 IU/L (range, 61-4279) in the MTX group. These authors concluded that low-dose oral MTX seems to be no more effective than placebo in women with ectopic pregnancy selected for expectant management.

The other study was a small clinical trial that compared prostaglandin therapy (local and systemic) with expectant management. A total of 23 patients with unruptured ectopic pregnancy and β-hCG levels < 2500 IU/L were included. The results showed that expectant management should only be recommended in a few selected cases, as it was significantly less successful than prostaglandin therapy (odds ratio [OR], 0.08; 95% confidence interval [CI], 0.02-0.39) [10].

All these data are also included in the 2007 Cochrane Database System Review [11]. More recent literature includes another clinical trial. The METEX study [12] is a multicenter, randomized clinical trial conducted in the Netherlands between April 2007 and January 2012. This study included 73 patients older than age 18 who were hemodynamically stable, had been diagnosed by ultrasound with ectopic pregnancy (ectopic ring or ectopic mass and/or fluid in the pouch of Douglas), and plateaued serum β-hCG levels < 1500 IU/L. Patients with signs of shock or fallopian tube rupture, an embryo with a positive heartbeat, or any contraindication for MTX were excluded. Patients who signed the informed consent were randomized to the expectant management group (32 patients) or a single intramuscular MTX injection of 1 mg/kg body weight (41 women) within 24 hours after randomization. The results showed no significant differences in cure rate between the two groups; 76% of patients treated with MTX (31/41) achieved negative β-hCG levels with no further medical action. In the expectant management group, 59% (19/32) progressed satisfactorily (relative risk [RR], 1.3; 95% CI, 0.9-1.8). Consequently, almost 60% of patients benefited from therapeutic abstention and from avoiding MTX, a potentially hazardous drug. According to the study authors, the main limitation was that no placebo group was included. However, there were no biases due to the use of strict inclusion criteria.

Ylöstalo [13] conducted a prospective study and found that approximately 20% of all tubal ectopic pregnancies will resolve spontaneously by tubal abortion into the abdominal cavity or by necrosis and cell reabsorption. The key is to clearly identify patients who will be cured with no pharmacologic or surgical intervention, in short, the group whose ectopic pregnancies are much less active. The problem, however, is that no pathognomonic signs exist to help select these patients. In view of the literature described and other recent articles [14], expectant management is a safe, acceptable, and effective treatment option of tubal ectopic pregnancy in cases of very less active ectopic pregnancies that can be defined using the following criteria:

- Clinical stability with no or minimal abdominal pain,
- No evidence of significant hemoperitoneum on ultrasound scan,
- Ectopic pregnancy measuring < 30 mm in mean diameter with no evidence of embryonic cardiac activity,
- Serum β-human chorionic gonadotropin (β-hCG) < 1500 IU/L, and
- Patient consent

Regarding expectant management and the issue of tubal patency and subsequent fertility, the 2007 Cochrane Database System Review [11] showed that there were no clinical trial data at the time. Tubal patency is defined as the passage of contrast material through the ipsilateral fallopian tube in hysterosalpingography or tubal chromopertubation in laparoscopy. Future fertility will depend on whether spontaneous intrauterine pregnancy is achieved in patients who wish to have offspring. To date, we have found no clinical trials, although there are descriptive observational studies that report their findings.

In 2007, Burster and Krotz [15] analyzed the data from previous studies to assess the impact of ectopic pregnancy treatment (laparoscopic salpingostomy, multiple-dose MTX, single-dose MTX, and expectant management) on subsequent fertility. They found no significant differences in reproductive results according to the treatment chosen. Among the 15 studies with expectant management, 76% (60/79) of patients showed tubal patency in the hysterosalpingography. A total of 57% (388/681) of patients subsequently achieved intrauterine pregnancy, and 13% (90/681) experienced another ectopic pregnancy.

Shortly afterwards, Helmy et al. [16] described a study that is the largest to date and included 444 patients (296 with salpingectomy; 134 with expectant management). Follow-up was possible in 173 (114 in the salpingectomy group; 59 in the expectant management group), and patients not desiring pregnancy were excluded. Spontaneous intrauterine pregnancy occurred in 41/49 (83.7%; 95% CI, 73.3%-94.2%) of patients managed expectantly and 62/97 (63.9%; 95% CI, 54.4-73.5%) in patients who underwent surgery (OR, 2.89; 95% CI, 1.22%-6.86%). There were no differences between the two groups in terms of the risk of a new ectopic pregnancy. These data showed that post-ectopic pregnancy fertility is similar between patients managed expectantly and patients treated by salpingectomy. However, the authors stated that the data should be interpreted with caution because the study was not a randomized trial.

Loss of fertility after an ectopic pregnancy is obviously related to tubal lesions and, in some cases, tubal occlusion. No data are available on hysterosalpingography findings after expectant management of ectopic pregnancy. However, according to the scientific literature to date, the effect of the various treatment strategies for ectopic pregnancy on subsequent fertility is still controversial. The main predictive factor for future fertility is the health of the contralateral fallopian tube. Hence, early diagnosis is essential for choosing the most conservative alternatives in the hope that tubal function and reproductive potential can be spared [17].

Medical Treatment

At present, medical treatment of ectopic pregnancy is synonymous with MTX. MTX is a folic acid antagonist that selectively inhibits the enzyme dihydrofolate reductase, thus preventing folates from being reduced to tetrahydrofolates. This metabolic event is not the only inherent event of the drug, as the agent also exerts an antiproliferative cellular effect via the polyglutamate chain. It acts by inhibiting thymidylate synthetase, stopping reactions key to *de novo* synthesis of purine and pyrimidine nucleotides and thus interrupting DNA and RNA synthesis. Because syncytiotrophoblast cells have strong metabolic activity, MTX has a trophic action on such cells and the drug works well, due to rich perfusion in the region.

MTX crosses the cell membrane weakly and requires a specific, active, and saturable transport mechanism to reach the cell cytoplasm. It leads to partial destruction of phase S populations inside the trophoblastic cell and is much more effective for logarithmic growth phases. This mechanism of action is responsible for regression of ectopic pregnancy.

The drug is readily absorbed in the gastrointestinal tract at low doses, but incompletely at higher doses, in which case parenteral administration is recommended. A total of 40% to 90% is excreted in urine as parent drug within 48 hours.

The toxic effects of MTX mainly affect the gastrointestinal tract and bone marrow and are usually reversible, although severe symptoms have been described. Obvious lesions in the intestinal epithelium will lead to nausea, abdominal pain, and bloody diarrhea. Bone marrow degeneration is seen in the circulating blood as pronounced leukopenia. There have also been reports of stomatitis, elevated liver enzymes, and at higher doses, anorexia, progressive weight loss, depression, and coma [18].

Medical treatment of ectopic pregnancy has been a real and safe alternative to classic laparoscopic surgery since 1982, when Tanaka [19] reported the first clinical case of a patient diagnosed with ectopic pregnancy and treated successfully with MTX. The patient was a 19-year-old Japanese woman with 7 weeks' amenorrhea who presented with pain in the left iliac fossa from 1 week earlier. The pelvic examination showed a tender mass on the left side of the uterine fundus. Urinary β-hCG levels were 64 000 IU/L.

Once left tubal ectopic pregnancy was diagnosed, laparotomy was performed, visualizing a left interstitial pregnancy of about 3x3 cm in the uterine angle, medial to the uterotubal junction. Because there was no blood in the abdominal cavity, the abdominal wall was closed and the surgery was ended. The patient immediately received 30 mg of intramuscular MTX, followed by 15 mg per day for 5 days. She required an additional two cycles of treatment to achieve urinary β-hCG levels below 40 IU/L. Based on the literature consulted, this was the first time that MTX was used to treat unruptured ectopic pregnancy and the article authors suggested that this option could be of interest in patients who wished to maintain their fertility and bear offspring.

In 1986 [20], the first case series was published, reporting on six patients diagnosed with ectopic pregnancy by laparoscopy and treated with four doses of intravenous MTX (1.0 mg/kg) followed by four doses of intramuscular leucovorin (0.1 mg/kg). Five of the six subjects experienced resolution of ectopic pregnancy without additional surgical treatment. One subject underwent salpingectomy following treatment. This preliminary experience showed that MTX may be an effective alternative for the treatment of early ectopic pregnancy.

In 1989, Stovall et al. [21] presented their series of 116 patients diagnosed with ectopic pregnancy by laparoscopy; 37 (46.3%) were selected for treatment with low-dose MTX and citrovorum factor, one of whom did not agree to the treatment. Treatment was successful in 94.4% (34/36) of patients and achieved complete resolution; the remaining two patients experienced complications with ectopic pregnancy rupture despite MTX. There were no major treatment-related complications, and 8.3% (3/36) of patients had minor side effects. Based on this study, MTX was considered a safe and effective treatment for the treatment of ectopic pregnancy and is presently considered the first-line drug.

A few years later, the same authors [22] described a prospective study that included 120 patients diagnosed with ectopic pregnancies with a diameter ≤ 3.5 cm. This key study introduced a single-dose regimen that is still used, namely, 50 mg/m^2 body surface area of single-dose intramuscular MTX, eliminating leucovorin rescue. Since the single dose was presented in 1993 until 2000, more than 700 cases treated with this therapeutic regimen had already been described, with a success rate of 87% (range, 75%-90%; reported in the meta-analysis by Morlock [23]).

One of the key aspects in medical treatment for ectopic pregnancy is to identify the ideal candidate to receive MTX. In 1991, Fernandez et al. [24] designed a study to investigate a pretherapy score that defined the indications of nonsurgical and surgical treatment in 61 patients diagnosed with ectopic pregnancy. The score used six criteria evaluated on a scale from 1 to 3: gestational age, β-hCG level, progesterone level, abdominal pain, hemoperitoneum volume, and hematosalpinx diameter (estimated by laparoscopy or transvaginal ultrasound). The authors found that a score ≤ 12 allowed 82% patients to be successfully managed without surgery. A score > 12 indicated that laparoscopic surgery may be more suitable. When ultrasound reveals an embryo heartbeat, medical treatment is always possible in patients with a score ≤ 12. Fernandez's score has been useful in clinical decision-making (Table 1) since 1991.

An ideal patient for MTX would have a Fernandez's score < 13 (criteria used in the 1990s) or "less active ectopic pregnancy" (criteria used at present), in short, situations in which the following criteria are met [25,26] (Table 2):

- Hemodynamic stability and no severe or persistent abdominal pain
- Low initial β-hCG concentration (<5000 IU/l)
- Small mass (< 4 cm) by transvaginal ultrasonography
- Unruptured mass
- No embryonic cardiac activity
- Certainty that there is no intrauterine pregnancy
- Willingness for follow-up
- No known sensitivity to MTX
- Normal baseline liver and renal function test results

When the patient to be treated with MTX is adequately selected, the success rate has been reported as 63% to 96.7% of cases [4] and according to the Practice Committee of the American Society for Reproductive Medicine [25], MTX represents first-line therapy for unruptured ectopic pregnancy that is diagnosed early.

Once MTX treatment has been decided, the ideal dose, follow-up, and route of administration must be defined.

Two MTX treatment regimens are commonly used at present: multiple dose and single dose (Table 3).

Table 1. Score for nonsurgical treatment, from Fernandez et al. [24]

Gestational age (weeks of amenorrhea)	> 8	7-8	< 7
β-hCG (IU/L)	< 1000	1000-5000	> 5000
Progesterone level (ng/mL)	< 5	5-10	> 10
Abdominal pain	Absent	Induced	Spontaneous
Hematosalpinx (cm)	< 1	1-3	> 3
Hemoperitoneum (mL)	0	1-100	> 100

Table 2. Selection of appropriate candidates for medical management of ectopic pregnancy [25,26]

Good Candidate	Poor Candidate	Contraindicated
Hemodynamically stable	High HCG (> 5000 IU/L)	Intrauterine pregnancy
No severe or persistent abdominal pain	Large mass (< 4 cm)	Evidence of immunodeficiency
Low β-HCG (< 5000 IU/L)	Embryonic cardiac activity present	Moderate to severe anemia, leucopenia or thrombocytopenia
Small mass (< 4 cm)	Significant abdominal pain	Sensitivity to MTX
Unruptured mass	Refusal to accept blood transfusion	Active pulmonary disease
No embryonic cardiac activity	Inability to participate in follow-up	Active peptic ulcer disease
Certainty that there is no intrauterine pregnancy		Clinically important liver impairment
Willingness for follow-up		Clinically important renal impairment
No known sensitivity to MTX		Breastfeeding

The multiple-dose protocol has been taken from the treatment of gestational trophoblast disease described by Goldstein in 1976 [27] and Bagshawe in 1989 [28]. These protocols include folinic acid (leucovarin) to attenuate the toxicity of chemotherapy. At present, the regimen used most often consists of four doses, which involve four MTX injections of 1 mg/kg/day, alternating every 24 hours with 0.1 mg/kg of leucovorin. Treatment is considered successful when β-hCG levels drop at least 15% from previous levels. β-hCG levels should be monitored weekly thereafter, until the results are negative [26]

Table 3. Methotrexate regimens used to treat ectopic pregnancy, taken from Bachman et al. [26]

Protocol (Dose)	MTX Dose	Regimen	β-hCG Measurement	Treatment Success	When to Administer Additional Dose
Multiple	1 mg/kg and 0.1 mg/kg leucovorin	Alternate daily doses of each	Days 0, 1, 3, 5, 7	β-hCG drops 15% from previous value	Second, third, or fourth dose given if β-hCG does not drop 15% from previous value. Maximum of 4 doses
Single	50 mg/m^2	Day 0	Days 0, 4, 7	β-hCG declines 15% between days 4 and 7	Second dose on day 7 if β-hCG does not drop 15%

The single-dose protocol was proposed by Stovall [22] in 1993 and consists of 50 mg/m^2 body surface area of intramuscular MTX as a single dose, eliminating leucovorin rescue therapy. Treatment success is defined as a drop of at least 15% in β-hCG levels between days 4 and 7, with patient follow-up thereafter consisting of weekly β-hCG testing until levels are undetectable. If the expected reduction is not achieved between day 4 and 7, the MTX dose should be repeated [26]. The data available in the literature do not clearly support either protocol. A meta-analysis [29] that included 1327 case reports from 26 papers was published in 2003, reporting an overall success rate for women treated with MTX for ectopic pregnancy was 89% (1181/1327), 88.1% for the single-dose regimen and 92.7% for the multiple dose regimen. The single dose was used much more frequently. The use of a single dose was associated with a significantly higher chance of failed medical management than the use of the multidose in both raw (OR, 1.71; 1.04, 2.82) and adjusted analyses (OR 4.74; 1.77, 12.62). The single-dose regimen was associated with fewer side effects (OR 0.44; 0.31, 0.63). Based on these data, the authors concluded that the multidose regimen was more effective than the single-dose regimen.

Later, the 2007 Cochrane Database System Review [11] included two clinical trials with a total of 159 patients diagnosed with ectopic pregnancy, in which the results showed no significant differences between the two treatment groups (OR, 0.89; 95% CI, 0.32-2.5). Mean serum β-hCG concentrations varied between 2230 to 2973 IU/L in the single-dose group (50 mg/m^2) and 2180 to 2244 IU/L in the multiple dose group (1 mg/kg). At present, the Practice Committee of the American Society for Reproductive Medicine [25] again recommends the multiple-dose protocol, as it has a lower failure rate than the single-dose MTX protocol.

Over time, a wide variety of MTX dosing routes has been tested, although all recent studies use the intramuscular route, either for a single-dose or multiple-dose regimen. There are several other possibilities:

- The oral route is debatable because, as stated earlier, MTX absorption in the gastrointestinal tract is limited at the therapeutic doses normally used [18]. Several published reports have addressed this issue. In 2002, Lipscomb et al., [30] used oral MTX given in two divided doses 2 hours apart at a dose of 60 mg/m^2 using 2.5-mg MTX tablets. In 86% of cases, the treatment was successful and, according to the authors, the oral route may be used, but intramuscular dosing would be recommended because it has few disadvantages.
- Local injection of the drug in the gestational sac has major advantages, as elevated MTX concentrations are achieved inside the ectopic pregnancy and general toxicity is reduced. If a laparoscopic approach is chosen [31], then the patient also runs the inherent risks of both this technique and the fluoroscopy-guided vaginal route [32], which makes it essential to locate the sac accurately. Additionally, the operator must have sufficient experience and adequate instruments.
- MTX instillation via hysteroscopic fallopian tube catheterization has also been tested, but requires skilled gynecologists [33].

The most innovative aspects related to MTX have been described by a working group at Tel Aviv University [34,35]. These authors propose a "watchful waiting" protocol for the management of patients diagnosed with ectopic pregnancy. The protocol was very conservative, as MTX was not immediately given to patients who met the criteria, but a "wait and see" attitude was taken according to β-hCG levels. A 15% drop in 24-hour β-hCG levels was assumed to indicate that the ectopic pregnancy had resolved spontaneously and no other action would be necessary. MTX was prescribed if

24-hour β-hCG levels rose 15% or more. For intermediate situations with β-hCG levels exhibiting a plateau or changes < 15%, watchful waiting was considered appropriate for up to 5 days and then MTX would be administered. The authors reported a study that included 1083 patients. In 674 (39.5%) of them, β-hCG levels dropped and the patient received no treatment. MTX treatment was successful in 87% of cases. The advantage of this protocol is that MTX alone is actually administered only to patients who need it and the side effects of the medication are prevented. MTX had a lower percentage of success, but this is certainly not accurate. Rather, the other papers also included patients who would heal alone, thus artificially raising the success rate. The most important disadvantage of this protocol is that it greatly lengthens the in-hospital time until a decision is made, but the authors stated that no economic assessment was performed.

Post-ectopic fertility in patients treated with MTX has not raised much interest among investigators. The Cochrane Database System Review [11] has reported that there were no conclusive data on subsequent fertility from clinical trials. The literature includes several observational studies from Auvergne et al. [36-38] and a few low-power clinical trials [39, 40] that found no statistically significant differences in subsequent fertility between the two conservative treatments (MTX and surgery with salpingostomy). The most recent, most well-designed study is the DEMETER randomized trial [41]. This was a randomized multicenter trial designed in 2003 to compare fertility in the first two years after ectopic pregnancy, according to type of treatment received (medical, conservative surgery, or radical surgery). Patients were divided into two groups: the first (n=207) included less active ectopic pregnancies (Fernandez's score < 13) and women were randomized to either conservative surgery plus MTX (n=97) or to MTX treatment (1 mg/kg IM) alone (n=110). After eliminating patients lost to follow-up, treatment failures, and patients not desiring pregnancy, the study saw no differences in the results. In the MTX treatment arm (87 women), 58 had intrauterine pregnancies and 8 had another ectopic pregnancy (12%). Among the conservative surgery group, 58/82 women had intrauterine pregnancies and 6/82 (9%) had another ectopic pregnancy. Based on these results, the authors concluded that post-ectopic pregnancy fertility did not vary according to the conservative treatment used.

Although post-ectopic fertility has traditionally been related to anatomic and functional fallopian tube integrity, new issues have been raised regarding the effect of MTX on the ovarian reserve. In recent years, this has been studied in patients who underwent *in vitro* fertilization and experienced ectopic pregnancy during that cycle and were treated with MTX.

Due to the antiproliferative effect of MTX, it has been speculated that the drug could act on the granulosa cells, preventing division and thus adversely affecting patients' ovarian reserve and reproductive future. In addition, if the woman underwent a cycle of *in vitro* fertilization and experienced ectopic pregnancy as the result, then MTX administration could hypothetically lead to greater damage due to a gonadotropin-induced increase in ovarian blood flow, thus producing inducing apoptosis in the granulosa cells and oocytes [42].

Boots et al. [42] specifically investigated these issues and concluded that MTX has no negative impact on later *in vitro* fertilization cycles, as patients treated with MTX have the same number of antral follicles, same FSH and retrieved oocyte levels, and overall good outcomes after treatment. The study was not free of limitations because it used a retrospective design with a small sample (n=66) and did not consider anti-müllerian hormone levels to assess ovarian response. Four previous studies [43-46] also investigated this hypothesis, observing the same results, and most showed no significant differences in either *in vitro* fertilization cycle parameters or outcomes.

Comparison between Medical Treatment (MTX) in a Single-Dose Regimen and Conservative Surgery

Success rates. A combination of three clinical trials [39,47,48] conducted in hemodynamically stable patients with small, unruptured ectopic pregnancies showed that a single dose of systemic MTX (50 mg/m^2 or 1 mg/kg IM) was significantly less successful than laparoscopic salpingostomy (RR, 0.82; 95% CI, 0.72-0.94). However, it is important is understand the indications for each therapeutic modality, and the Practice Committee of the American Society for Reproductive Medicine [25] has concluded that post-treatment success rates are comparable for medical therapy and conservative surgical treatment. Therefore, both conservative surgery and medical therapy may be viewed as appropriate first-line therapies in many early unruptured ectopic pregnancies.

Recovery time. Recovery time is the time to negative serum β-hCG levels after ectopic pregnancy and varies from 20 to 31 days. Because medical treatment can fail due to trophoblast persistence after salpingostomy (particularly if MTX is not administered postoperatively), β-hCG levels must be monitored until the result is < 2 IU/L [4]. Several clinical trials have compared the recovery time after conservative surgery and MTX. In 1998, Saraj et al. [47] presented a prospective randomized clinical trial that evaluated resolution of serum β-hCG and progesterone levels in patients (n=75) with ectopic pregnancy who received single-dose intramuscular MTX (n=38) and compared it to patients undergoing laparoscopic salpingostomy (n=37). The mean time for β-hCG concentrations to drop to < 15 mIU/mL was significantly shorter for laparoscopic salpingostomy than for MTX: 20.2 ± 2.7 and 27.2 ± 2.3 days, respectively ($P < .05$). Colarcurci et al. [49] conducted a similar study; in which group 1 included 15 patients treated with linear salpingostomy and group 2 included 15 patients treated with MTX. The time to resolution was 33.6 ± 6.6 days in group 1 and 31.5 ± 7.8 days in group 2, differences that were not statistically meaningful. Therefore, the authors concluded that the outcomes were comparable to those seen with laparoscopic treatment and suggested that β-hCG becomes negative regardless of type of treatment and residual trophoblast. In recent years, the DEMETER study [41] also found that the recovery time is shorter in the conservative surgery group plus MTX than the group that received MTX alone, and that the differences were statistically significant. These studies appear to demonstrate that recovery time is shorter in patients who have undergone laparoscopic surgery; however, in my opinion, it is even more important to monitor β-hCG levels until they are negative.

Cost. In 2001, Sowter et al. [50] presented a study that compared the direct and indirect costs of single-dose systemic MTX with laparoscopic surgery for unruptured ectopic pregnancy. These authors performed a cost minimization study performed with a randomized trial and included 62 women with ectopic pregnancy randomized to either single-dose MTX (50 mg/m^2) or laparoscopic surgery. The economic evaluation showed systemic MTX therapy in eligible ectopic pregnancy patients led to significantly reduced direct costs. Most likely, indirect costs to women and their caregivers were lowered only when pretreatment serum β-hCG levels were 1500 IU/L. Recently, the Practice Committee of the American Society for Reproductive Medicine [25] also concluded that medical therapy seems to be more cost-effective than surgery except when initial β-hCG level are high or an embryo heartbeat is observed.

Physical and psychological functioning. In 1998, Nieuwkerk et al. [51] undertook a multicenter randomized clinical trial to compare patients' health-related quality of life after systemic MTX therapy versus laparoscopic salpingostomy for tubal pregnancy. Patients were given standard health-related quality of life questionnaires at baseline and then 2 days, 2 weeks, 4 weeks, and 16 weeks after laparoscopy to confirm ectopic pregnancy. Systemic MTX affected patients' health-related quality of life more adversely than laparoscopic salpingostomy, and it was concluded that due consideration should be given to this impact during the decision-making process in tubal pregnancy. Another study published in 2001 [48] reported that physical functioning was significantly better in women treated with MTX than in women who underwent laparoscopic surgery ($P < .01$) but found no differences in psychological functioning.

Women's preferences. There is scant literature on women's preferences for ectopic pregnancy treatment. However, in 1998 a report was published on a study [52] that investigated patient preferences for systemic MTX versus and laparoscopic salpingostomy for tubal pregnancy. The authors concluded that most patients would prefer systemic MTX as part of a completely nonsurgical management strategy. Only a few patients felt that tubal patency was key to the decision, and some patients stated that they would never choose systemic MTX. Patient preferences regarding systemic MTX are highly individualistic and should be considered when deciding on treatment. These preferences will basically depend on the treatment options offered by the patient's gynecologist and the doctor-patient relationship. A more recent paper published in 2013 investigated patient satisfaction, but only included patients who underwent surgery [53]. However, its conclusions can be extrapolated to medical treatment, as good doctor-patient communication and complete, detailed and understandable information will help to improve the clinical picture substantially.

Conservative Surgery (Salpingotomy)

Surgical treatment is reserved for "active ectopic pregnancies" when the fallopian tube is either ruptured or about to rupture in hemodynamically unstable patients. The decision to perform conservative or radical surgery is usually made during the procedure and depends mainly on the patient's history (salpingectomy is indicated in the case of ipsilateral recurrence), the appearance and condition of the contralateral fallopian tube, and the presence of any bleeding. If the fallopian tube is ruptured, radical surgery should not be routinely performed unless hemostasis is expected to be difficult. Fallopian tube removal will most certainly be the best choice than a tube-sparing procedure if it is in poor condition [4].

In both conservative and radical surgery, the surgical approach is not usually questioned. Laparoscopy is clearly the treatment of choice compared to laparotomy, and its advantages include a shorter hospital stay, lower costs, decreased morbidity (mainly postoperative pain), shorter surgical time, more limited blood loss during surgery, and fewer postoperative adhesions [54]. Laparoscopic surgery is safe even in cases of hypovolemic shock, provided that there is adequate laparoscopic material, a skilled nursing team, and surgeons with advanced laparoscopic skills. Most importantly, the surgeon must be familiar with the latest laparoscopic techniques and exercise clinical judgment in choosing the best management strategy and understanding one's limitations. Patients must be stabilized before surgery, if necessary by intravenous colloid infusion or blood transfusion. A bladder catheter should be inserted, and diuresis and vital signs should be monitored, possibly by invasive hemodynamic techniques. Once the patient is stable, the surgery can begin. It is crucial for the anesthesiologist to agree on the surgeon's choice to undertake laparoscopic surgery [55]. It has been speculated that in the case of active bleeding, creation of pneumoperitoneum with a Verres needle could lengthen the time to hemostasis control. Several classic studies [56] showed that entry via direct trocar insertion is possible without a higher number of major complications and with a shorter time for the entry technique (2.2 minutes versus 5.9 minutes for the direct insertion and Verres needle techniques, respectively). Therefore, in patients with bleeding ectopic pregnancy where time is critical, direct entry with the trocar may be recommended. The next point to consider in cases of hemoperitoneum is pelvic organ visualization. Consequently, routine placement of an intrauterine manipulator (except in cases of heterotopic pregnancy) will facilitate fallopian tube exposure and help identify the bleeding site, although increased intra-abdominal pressure from pneumoperitoneum could falsely occlude the bleeding point. It is essential to have appropriate material available, particularly a bipolar electrocoagulation system and a 10-mm suction-irrigation system [55]. In view of all these recommendations, laparoscopy is safer than laparotomy, even in critical situations.

Laparoscopic salpingostomy was first mentioned in 1967 by Manhes and Bruhat [57], and essentially the same surgical technique is still used at present. The hemoperitoneum must be evacuated to avoid hindering endoscopic vision, and preventive hemostasis must be achieved by instilling a vasoconstrictor agent at the site of the ectopic pregnancy and at the two ends of the vascular hila below the fallopian tube to prevent both intraoperative and postoperative bleeding. The fallopian tube is then approached and salpingotomy is performed by electrosection (scissors could also be used to prevent tissue damage), making a millimetric, longitudinal incision at the antimesenteric border of the fallopian tube, with the incision made at the junction of the inner third with the outer two thirds of the hematosalpinx. The trophoblast is then aspirated through the salpingotomy. The suction tube diameter must be large enough to exert proper traction and allow complete removal of the material. Traction must be progressive to avoid breaking up the trophoblast. The intervention is completed with hemostasis control of the fallopian tube; slight pressure on the fallopian tube is simplest, as it is agreed that electrocoagulation (even when bipolar) should be avoided to prevent irreversible fallopian tube lesions. Salpingotomy suture is not necessary. Adequate lavage of the region is necessary to remove any trophoblastic residue in the abdominal cavity. The procedure does not require specialized surgical material, but it is extremely important to use a large-diameter aspirator and unipolar electrocautery unit. The Triton multipurpose device invented by Manhes combines electrocoagulation, aspiration, and lavage in the same instrument, a tool that is highly advisable but not essential [58].

Four factors are decisive when choosing between conservative and radical surgery: surgical morbidity, risk of failure, desire for pregnancy, and prognosis of fertility, which includes the probability of intrauterine pregnancy and the risk of recurrence of ectopic pregnancy [59].

- ***Surgical morbidity.*** As we explained previously, both techniques can be safely performed with adequate laparoscopic equipment, a skilled nursing team, and surgeons with advanced laparoscopic skills. Firstly, the surgeon must consider the ectopic pregnancy site: in interstitial ectopic pregnancies, medical treatment with MTX is recommended but conservative treatment must be avoided if surgery is needed. Secondly, hemostasis is a major consideration, as salpingectomy becomes essential if vasoconstrictors are not available or bleeding cannot be controlled. Thirdly, the fallopian tube must be in good condition, and salpingectomy is preferable if the fallopian tube is unlikely to heal properly [60].
- ***Risk of failure.*** The persistence of ectopic trophoblastic tissue is one of the main complications of conservative surgery and the main reason why a second operation is sometimes needed. Incomplete trophoblast ablation will lead to progressive encysted hematocele with persistently elevated β-hCG levels. The first case of trophoblast persistence was described by Kelly et al. in 1979 [61], and later literature contains many reports. A meta-analysis [11] of randomized clinical trials showed that laparoscopic salpingostomy is associated with a high probability of persistence of trophoblastic tissue (3%-20% of cases). Similar data have been recently reported by the ESEP study

[62], an open-label, multicenter randomized controlled trial designed to determine if fertility outcomes improve after salpingotomy versus salpingectomy. This trial reported trophoblast persistence in 7% (14/215) of patients who underwent conservative surgery, compared with < 1% (1/231) in the radical surgery group, a difference that was significant. In addition, 2% (5/215) of patients required repeat laparoscopy and salpingectomy due to trophoblast persistence. Based on these findings, the technique should be abandoned and salpingectomy should be performed if any of the risk factors for persistence are present: 1) large ectopic pregnancy [63], which requires salpingectomy (the reports vary, but conservative treatment is generally not recommended for a diameter > 3-5 cm); 2) poor fallopian tube access, with salpingostomy not recommendable in cases of obesity or peritubal adhesions; 3) β-hCG levels > 8000 IU/L, making salpingostomy not advisable [64]; and 4) poor condition of the fallopian tube, with salpingectomy usually indicated when the fallopian tube is significantly injured. These are recommendations only, however, and not absolute contraindications. The surgeon should assess each individual carefully and decide based on these criteria and his or her experience.

- In order to minimize the possibility of trophoblast persistence after salpingostomy, the option of associating systemic MTX after surgery has been repeatedly considered, although routine use is still debated. A clinical trial in 129 patients who underwent linear salpingostomy was presented in 1997. This trial included two groups: a control group of 62 women who underwent surgery alone and a prophylaxis group of 54 women treated with a single dose of MTX 1 mg/kg intramuscularly within 24 hours after surgery. Persistent ectopic pregnancy was defined as a rise in serum β-hCG levels or a decline of less than 20% between two consecutive measurements taken three days apart. Ten women had persistent ectopic pregnancy, one (1.9%) in the prophylaxis group and nine (14.5%) among the controls, a difference that was statistically significant ($P < .05$). The RR of developing persistent ectopic pregnancy after prophylactic MTX was 0.13 (95% confidence interval 0.02, 0.97). Mild side effects were reported by three (5.5%) women after MTX, but resolved spontaneously. Based on these results, the authors concluded that, "the incidence of persistent ectopic pregnancy was significantly reduced after a single prophylactic dose of systemic MTX administered postoperatively. This regimen is safe and can be used to decrease the extent of postoperative monitoring after conservative treatment of unruptured ectopic pregnancy" [65]. However, due to the high risk of adverse reactions with MTX, the Cochrane Database System Review [11] authors do not recommend the routine use of systemic MTX after laparoscopic salpingostomy; the adverse effects reported are mainly asymptomatic elevation of liver enzymes, with rare cases of drug-induced hepatitis (1%). Recently, the DEMETER study also confirmed that postoperative MTX injection significantly reduces the persistence of trophoblast. In 2013, the Practice Committee of the American Society for Reproductive Medicine [25] concluded that postoperative, prophylactic, single-dose systemic MTX may reduce the incidence of persistent ectopic pregnancy after salpingostomy. Therefore, the issue of whether routine postoperative MTX injection is safe and cost-effective still requires a definitive answer, particularly when MTX use could simplify the subsequent follow-up necessary. Because the likelihood of failures is very low, β-hCG levels can be tested one month later [4].

- ***Desire for offspring***. If pregnancy is not desired, then radical treatment with salpingectomy, possibly associated with contralateral sterilization, is clearly indicated [66].
- ***Prognosis of fertility.*** It has classically been considered that organ-sparing requires conservative surgery, although this is not an absolute necessity in the case of paired organs. The prognosis of fertility is studied based on two variables:
  - ✓ *Probability of subsequent intrauterine pregnancy*. The literature reports are inconsistent. Some classic studies apparently found no differences between conservative and radical techniques [67-69], whereas others report the rate of intrauterine pregnancies achieved was higher after salpingostomy [70-72]. However, these series were observational studies, and in 2009, the Cochrane Database System Review [11] found no conclusive data related to subsequent fertility. In 2012, the findings were presented for another observational study that included 164 patients from the Auvergne Registry who had been diagnosed with ectopic pregnancy between 1992 and 2008. The 24-month cumulative rate of intrauterine pregnancy was 67% after salpingectomy and 76% after salpingostomy. Intrauterine pregnancy was less likely to occur after radical treatment than after conservative treatments

in univariate analyses. In multivariate analyses, however, the intrauterine pregnancy rate was significantly lower when patients were > 35 years old or had a history of infertility or tubal disease. In these patients, the intrauterine pregnancy rate was significantly more common after conservative treatment than after salpingectomy. Consequently, these authors [36] defend the use of conservative surgery whenever possible. Most recently, as stated earlier, two multicenter randomized clinical trials were conducted to compare fertility after ectopic pregnancy according to the type of treatment received. The first was called the DEMETER study, after the Greek fertility goddess known as Heratas, and was designed in 2003; its second arm was proposed to compare conservative surgery plus MTX (101 patients) to radical surgery (98 patients). Once the analysis excluded patients lost to follow-up or who did not desire pregnancy, the rate of pregnancy was similar in both groups. The authors followed patients for 2 years after treatment (radical versus conservative), but found no significant differences in subsequent fertility [41]. The ESPE study [73] was published the same year and showed that salpingotomy did not improve cumulative rates of ongoing pregnancy due to natural conception in women with a history of tubal pregnancy and a healthy contralateral tube. The median time to ongoing pregnancy by natural conception was 20 months (95% CI, 17-23) after salpingotomy and 26 months (95% CI, 15-37) after salpingectomy. The cumulative rate of ongoing pregnancy by natural conception after 36 months was 60.7% after salpingotomy and 56.2% after salpingectomy. Therefore, both clinical trials had similar findings and conclusions, namely, that salpingectomy is preferable to salpingostomy in women with a healthy contralateral fallopian tube (the ESEP study excluded patients with contralateral tubal disease whereas the DEMETER study did not).

✓ *Risk of recurrence.* The main argument for radical treatment is the need to eliminate recurrences, but the literature indicates that this is a false premise. Although this was already seen in previous observational studies, the DEMETER study [41] showed that the recurrence rate in arm 2 (conservative surgery plus MTX versus radical surgery) was similar in both groups; in particular, recurrence was 8% (4/63) in the salpingostomy group and 12.5%

> (6/66) in the salpingectomy group. These results were also reported by the ESEP study [73], which observed recurrence in 8% (18/215) of new ectopic pregnancies in the salpingotomy group and 5% (12/231) in the salpingectomy group (nonsignificant differences). Therefore, unilateral salpingectomy does not prevent the recurrence of ectopic pregnancy.

No strict recommendations have been made, and the latest data are conflicting. According to the EPSE study, salpingectomy is preferred over salpingostomy in patients with ectopic pregnancy and a healthy contralateral fallopian tube. In contrast, D'Hooghe and Tomassetti [74] critique the EPSE study, proposing that if surgical treatment is necessary, salpingostomy should also be offered even if the contralateral fallopian tube is normal, particularly in women older than age 35 years or with a history of sterility. In women younger than 35 years with a normal contralateral fallopian tube and no history of sterility or tubal disease, the decision should be made carefully by the patient and her gynecologist, based on his or her surgical experience and the potential benefits and risks of each technique.

Radical Surgery (Salpingectomy)

In 1987, Dubbuisson et al. [75] reported the first laparoscopic salpingectomy performed to treat ectopic pregnancy. These authors presented 100 consecutive cases of patients diagnosed with ampullary ectopic pregnancy, with a laparotomy reconversion rate of 2%. At the time, they described the technique as rapid, simple and virtually free of complications.

The description of the surgical technique is still practically the same [76]. The hemoperitoneum should be aspirated if necessary to achieve satisfactory exposure of the affected fallopian tube and assess the ectopic pregnancy and entire pelvic cavity (size, rupture or nonrupture, presence of adhesions, condition of contralateral fallopian tube, etc.), with adhesiolysis performed, if necessary. Retrograde salpingectomy can then be started. The procedure is started by clamping the fallopian tube in place at its isthmic portion at a distance of 1.5 cm from the uterine horn, thus achieving good exposure of the fallopian tube isthmus and mesosalpinx. Bipolar electrocoagulation is used to coagulate the mesosalpinx and its posterior cut, until the proximal portion of the fallopian tube is reached (at a distance of 1-2 cm from the uterine horn). The fallopian tube is then electrocoagulated with bipolar energy and cutting.

Once the fallopian tube is sectioned, the tube must be extracted either by an endoscopic sac introduced over a 12-mm trocar or by direct removal through one of the suprapubic routes, size permitting. The surgery is completed once hemostasis has been confirmed and the abdominal and pelvic cavity has been carefully washed.

Salpingectomy is performed conventionally using multi-pore laparoscopy (MPLS); placement of a 10-mm trocar in the umbilical incision for the chamber and at least two 5-mm accessory trocars inserted into the left and right lower quadrants (a third suprapubic trocar will normally be introduced). Recent studies present the possibility of single-port laparocopic salpingectomy (SPLS) for the treatment of ectopic pregnancy [77]. This is laparoscopic access through a single 15-mm umbilical trocar (instead of the three or four accesses in conventional surgery), which is rapidly being developed in all surgical fields (due to the advantages of minimally invasive access) and may represent next-generation endoscopic surgery. The multichannel laparoscopic access device allows multiple instruments to be introduced simultaneously through a single incision and ensures that pneumoperitoneum is maintained regardless of whether these instruments are inserted or not. The laparoscopic instruments used were similar to those employed in conventional laparoscopy; however, the instruments are straight and stiff, which may hinder the visual field during surgery and allow them to cross. Kim et al. [77] have presented a retrospective analysis of 63 patients with tubal pregnancy who underwent SPLS and 71 patients who underwent conventional MPLS. The authors found no differences in surgical time and complications between both groups. In addition, SPLS has the advantages of incision-free surgery. Its main limitation is that this single-port technique requires time for surgeon training and requires sufficient surgical skill. Nonetheless, SPLS may be an effective alternative to MPLS.

The indications, advantages and disadvantages of this technique have already been discussed in the previous section.

New Pharmacologic Strategies

The new pharmacologic strategies are hypothetically intended to enhance MTX efficacy and increase the percentage of ectopic pregnancies that can be safely treated medically, thus avoiding surgery. According to Jurkovic and Wilkinson [78], MTX has a limited role because not more than 25% to 30% of ectopic pregnancies meet the criteria to be safely treated using a medical strategy. Therefore, any new therapeutic agent able to raise the success rate would increase the percentage of ectopic pregnancies cured with no need for surgery.

These new drugs (mifepristone and gefitinib) would be indicated in hemodynamically stable patients with active ectopic pregnancies when the fallopian tube is not yet ruptured but the risk is high. Patients could benefit if they do not fully meet the treatment criteria for MTX (eg, ectopic pregnancies with very high β-hCG levels, very large ectopic pregnancies, or live embryos), in short, if they have signs indicating that an ectopic pregnancy is in progress.

At present, there is considerably more experience with mifepristone. Molecularly, this drug selectively occupies and competes with the endogenous progesterone receptor, thus destroying trophoblastic and decidual tissue, lowering luteinizing-hormone levels, and blocking the corpora lutea, which leads to embryo necrosis and abortion [79]. The drug was first used in the past century as sole treatment for ectopic pregnancy, but the results were not encouraging and the few published case studies and small case series report poor success rates. In 1998, two methodologically well-designed clinical trials [80, 81] that combined MTX and mifepristone were published almost simultaneously and led to abandonment of the idea that success could be obtained with mifepristone alone. Mifepristone was the first drug with antiprogestogen efficacy; the hypothesis was that its effect on ectopic pregnancy might not be strong enough to achieve resolution, but that the agent could have important adverse effects on the development of the ectopic trophoblast. Hence, combining MTX with mifepristone would be another medical alternative for ectopic pregnancy that would be more rapid, more effective, and offer a lower risk of side effects.

Gazvani et al. [80], a group at the Liverpool Women's Hospital, published the first paper in July 1998 and presented 50 patients diagnosed with tubal ectopic pregnancy by laparoscopy. Women were randomized to receive a single intramuscular injection of 50 mg/m^2 MTX alone or a single 600-mg dose of oral mifepristone in combination with the same dose of MTX. Both protocols successfully achieved resolution of unruptured ectopic pregnancy (18/25 in the MTX group; 22/25 in the mifepristone-MTX group) following the initial intervention. A second injection was needed in 4/25 (16%) cases in the MTX group and 1/25 (4%) case in the mifepristone-MTX group. Full resolution was achieved in 22/25 and 23/25 cases, respectively. Moreover, resolution of unruptured ectopic pregnancy was faster in women given MTX + mifepristone than in women given MTX alone ($P = .01$). The effect of MTX-mifepristone was stronger in women with higher β-hCG levels (> 423 IU/L).

The authors concluded that the MTX-mifepristone combination was a good alternative to single-dose MTX, although they underscored the need for larger studies to confirm if this treatment option would also be better for reproductive function-sparing and fewer complications.

In September 1998, Perdu et al. [81] presented their preliminary results from a nonrandomized phase II study which included all patients with ectopic pregnancy in progress who met the criteria for medical management. Treatment consisted of 50 mg/m^2 of intramuscular MTX and 600 mg of oral mifepristone, compared with a previous group that received only 50 mg/m^2 of intramuscular MTX. Failure was observed in 1/30 patients who received the combination and 11/42 patients treated with MTX alone. The authors concluded that the mifepristone-MTX combination lowered the risk of failed medical treatment in ectopic pregnancy. In addition, β-hCG levels on day 4 were lower among patients treated with the mifepristone-MTX combination, which would suggest that trophoblast lysis was more rapid in that group. Therefore, faster action would lower the risk of fallopian tube rupture and hemoperitoneum. In fact, an earlier study [82] had already found pronounced trophoblastic necrosis in the histologic study of samples taken from ectopic pregnancies treated with mifepristone. Lastly, the authors pointed out the need for a new, prospective, multicenter, double-blind, randomized study to compare MTX and mifepristone with MTX and placebo.

In the early 21st century (2003), research continued on the possible benefits of the mifepristone-MTX association, as Perdú et al. [81] had previously suggested. Rozenberg et al. [83] presented the first prospective, multicenter, randomized clinical trial in patients with tubal ectopic pregnancy to compare the efficacy of MTX and mifepristone (600 mg PO, single-dose) versus MTX and placebo. From an initial population of 597 patients diagnosed with ectopic pregnancy at 18 participating sites between October 1999 and April 2001, 212 patients were finally included in the study. Among these women, 113/212 (53.3%) were included in the MTX-mifepristone group and 99/212 (46.7%) in the MTX-placebo group. In both groups, the basic characteristics at baseline (age, gravidity, parity, gestational age, β-hCG at inclusion, progesterone, adnexal mass, size, gestational cardiac activity, hemoperitoneum, and volume) were similar. The main finding of this study was that there were no statistically significant differences between the two groups. The overall success rate was 77.1% (162/210) for medical treatment: 79.6% (90/113) for the MTX-mifepristone group and 74.2% (72/97) for the MTX-placebo combination. Nevertheless, patients with high progesterone levels (> 10 ng/mL) had better outcomes with the MTX-mifepristone combination than with MTX-placebo. In particular, both groups achieved similar outcomes in patients with low progesterone levels (success rate of 76.5% in the mifepristone arm and 80% in the placebo arm). In the case of high progesterone levels (> 10 ng/mL), the success rate was 83.3% (15/18) in the mifepristone group and only 38.5% (5/13) in the placebo group. The authors concluded that the MTX-mifepristone combination should be reserved for ectopic pregnancies with high progesterone levels, and that another randomized clinical trial should be performed in this population.

Elevated serum progesterone concentrations in ectopic pregnancy simply indicate the presence of an active corpora lutea and a pregnancy in progress [84]. Therefore, particularly in these cases, mifepristone will have the added benefit of a luteolytic effect, facilitating the necrosis of trophoblastic tissue [85,86]. In summary, based on the literature review, mifepristone plays an important role as MTX co-adjuvant in the treatment of unruptured tubal ectopic pregnancy in patients with elevated progesterone levels (> 10 ng/mL), given its luteolytic effect.

Scientific research has continued from 2003 to date, but there have been no new contributions. Mifepristone has been investigated in many studies (Table 4), case reports, systematic reviews, clinical trials, etc., and the MTX-mifepristone combination is currently accepted for the treatment of unruptured tubal ectopic pregnancies in progress with high progesterone levels, in short, in "active ectopic pregnancies" (but always individualized), as it has been shown to be a safe, effective therapy with few side effects. This has been the case, even though a 2005 U.S. Food and Drug Administration (FDA) publication [87] stated that "mifepristone is not effective for the treatment of ectopic pregnancy." The conclusions drawn from the literature are clear, although some authors [88] have already addressed the potential medical-legal repercussions of these declarations. Current research is focusing on the role of gefitinib in the management of ectopic pregnancy [89-91]. Gefitinib is a small molecule that selectively inhibits tyrosine kinase in the epidermal growth factor receptor. Epidermal growth factor (EGF) is a protein substance that, together with hormones and neurotransmitters, plays an important role in intercellular communication and stimulates cell proliferation by regulating the cell cycle, maintaining cell survival, stimulating cell migration, cell differentiation, and even apoptosis. It has mytogenic capacity on a wide variety of epithelial cells, hepatocytes, and fibroblasts. This activity is important in wound healing, a context in which EGF is secreted by macrophages, keratinocytes, and other inflammatory cells migrating to the injured area and widely distributed in tissue secretions and fluids.

Table 4. Studies of Mifepristone and the MTX-mifepristone combination in the treatment of unruptured tubal ectopic pregnancies in progress with high progesterone levels

Author	Year	Study Type	Drugs	MFP Dose	Outcomes Success Rate	Conclusion
Sowter and Farquhar [92]	2004	Review article				MFP is another therapeutic agent
Garbin O et al. [93]	2004	Clinical trial	MTX-MFP MTX-Placebo	600 mg, oral	MTX-MFP: 79.6% (90/113). For $P > 10$ ng/L, 83.3% (15/18) MTX-Placebo: 74.2% (72/97). For $P > 10$ ng/L, 38.5% (5/13)	MTX-MFP could be reserved for ectopic pregnancies associated with high serum progesterone concentrations
Li and Quan [94]	2004	Clinical trial	MTX-MFP-CLMTX-CL	75 mg, oral, twice daily for 3 days	MTX-MFP-CL: 92.2% (94/102) MTX-CL: 81.4% $P < .05$	MTX-MFP-CL is safe and effective in the treatment of tubal ectopic pregnancy, with no obvious side effects
Lozeau and Potter [82]	2005	Review article				MFP is another therapeutic agent
Song HD et al. [95]	2006	Meta-analysis (23 randomized controlled trials involving 1706 patients)	MTX-MFP MTX			MTX-MFP may be effective with good safety and minimal side effects; however, this conclusion should be confirmed by double-blind randomized controlled trials with a larger sample size and more rigorous trial design.
Hajenius PJ et al. [11]	2007	*Cochrane Library* Review				Includes the studies and conclusions of Gazvani [80] in 1998 and Rozenberg [83] in 2003
Veena P [96]	2011	Case study	MTX-MFP	600 mg, oral	100% (1/1)	Larger case series are needed to establish the safety and efficacy of this treatment
Varma and Gupta [97]	2012	Systematic review				Includes the studies and conclusions of Perdu [81] in 1998, Gazvani [80] in 1998, Rozenberg [83] in 2003, and Hajenius [11] in 2007

Abbreviations: CL, calcium leucovorin; MFP, mifepristone; MTX, methotrexate; P, progesterone.

EGF works at very low concentrations, acting through its cell receptor in the cell membrane by transmitting the signal inward from the outside, in order to activate a signal cascade that ends with activation of one or more genes. EGF receptor (EGFR) belongs to a superfamily of receptors located in the plasma membrane that has inherent tyrosine kinase activity. EGF and its receptors are also expressed in carcinogenic cells and represent an important factor for increased tumor cell growth, apoptosis blockade, increased production of angiogenic factors, and to facilitate metastasis processes.

Gefitinib selectively inhibits tyrosine kinase activity, which means that EGFR fails to trigger intracellular transduction signals, cell growth is blocked, and apoptosis is induced. This mechanism of action is responsible for the efficacy of the drug in treating patients with non-small cell lung cancer or breast cancer.

Placental tissue has been found to strongly express EGFR compared to other nonmalignant tissues. Moreover, its activation promotes cytotrophoblastic mobility, blocks programmed trophoblastic cell death, and rescues the placenta from apoptosis when exposed to hypoxia or toxic stimuli. By blocking EGFR, gefitinib hypothetically induces cell death of ectopic trophoblastic tissue. This is the theoretical base for the possible efficacy of the drug in the treatment of ectopic pregnancy, which is currently being investigated by a multicenter working group [89-91].

The initial results from the Nilsson et al. [89] group were obtained using an animal model. These researchers investigated the effects of the gefitinib-MTX combination on three types of placental cells *in vitro*: JEG3 cells (choriocarcinoma cell line, which models trophoblast cells), BeWo cells (choriocarcinoma cell line, which models syncytiotrophoblasts, the cell layer covering the placental surface), and cells isolated from the first-trimester. The group investigated whether combining these agents was more potent in blocking the activation of EFGR and causing apoptosis than either agent alone. Lastly, they examined the effects of adding gefitinb to placental tissue in two animal models. The authors showed that EGFR was highly expressed on the surface of placental tissues from ectopic pregnancies, that the gefitinib-MTX combination potently induces placental cell death, and that this observation was seen in three placental cell types. The combination of both drugs causes greater placenta cell apoptosis compared to a single drug. Therefore, they conclude that the gefitinib-MTX combination may be a promising strategy for medical treatment of ectopic pregnancy. The limitation of this study is that there are no animal models specifically for ectopic pregnancy. However, it was possible to conduct the study using primary placental cells from first-trimester placenta of aborting patients, despite the difficulty entailed in obtaining this type of cell. In any case, this line of research is still open.

In October 2013, the same investigators [90] presented a phase I, single-arm (nonrandomized), open-label study conducted to determine the safety, tolerability, and efficacy of gefitinib plus MTX to treat ectopic pregnancy. They included 12 patients who had been diagnosed with ectopic pregnancy, were hemodynamically stable, had β-hCG levels below 3000 IU/L, a minimal amount of free pelvic fluid, a gestational sac smaller than 4 cm and with no embryonic cardiac activity, and normal blood counts and liver/renal panels. The study excluded women who had a history of significant respiratory, gastrointestinal or dermatologic illness or who were of Japanese ethnicity, due to the high incidence of pulmonary disease among Japanese women. The women received 50 mg/m^2 intramuscular MTX on day 1 and daily oral 250 mg gefitinib using a dose-escalation protocol. The first three participants received 250 mg gefitinib on day 1, the next three received 250 mg per day of gefitinib for 3 days, and the last six participants received 250 mg per day of gefitinib for 7 days. Based on the study results, combination treatment did not cause significant toxicities. The most common side effects were transient acneiform rash in 67% (8/12) and diarrhea in 42% (5/12), known side effects of gefitinib. There was no clinical or biochemical evidence of serious pulmonary, renal, hepatic, or hematologic toxicity. Regarding the efficacy of the combined treatment, ectopic pregnancy was resolved in 10/12 (83%) patients. The investigators created a subgroup of six patients with β-hCG levels of 1000-3000 IU/L and compared it with a historic cohort of 71 women with the same characteristics who had been treated with MTX alone. In the combination treatment subgroup, β-hCG levels dropped more rapidly (34% less time to cure) than in the MTX cohort. The authors concluded that the gefitinib-MTX combination is potentially more effective than MTX alone and suggest that the combined treatment could be useful in other trophoblastic growth disorders, such as persistent gestational trophoblastic disease or placenta accreta, or in the treatment of nontubal ectopic pregnancies (eg, cervix, interstitial, caesarean scar), which are potentially serious situations. The main limitation of this study is the low number (12) of patients included and the fact that the trial had only one arm, as a second arm with patients of the same characteristics but treated with MTX alone should have been included.

The same working group [91] is currently conducting a simple-arm, open-label, multicenter phase II trial to evaluate the efficacy and side effects of a combination of gefitinib and MTX to treat tubal ectopic pregnancies. The study included 28 patients with β-hCG levels of 1000-10000 IU/L, using the same exclusion criteria as for phase I. Patients will be treated with single-dose intramuscular MTX (50 mg/m^2) injection with seven daily doses of oral gefitinib (250 mg). The primary endpoint is to determine the cure rate of patients (avoiding surgery), and the secondary endpoints are to confirm the time to resolution (and compare it with the historic MTX cohort) and to determine the safety and tolerability of the combined treatment. The authors expect a success rate of at least 90%. The results have still not been published; however, the authors reiterate the fact that this treatment is not yet approved.

In conclusion, the range of therapeutic options for ectopic pregnancy is extremely broad and varied. The right decision for each case must be made will depend on the individual characteristics of each patient, each gynecologist, and each facility.

References

[1] Chang J, Elam-Evans LD, Berg CJ, Herndon J, Flowers L, Seed KA, Syverson CJ. Pregnancy-related mortality surveillance--United States, 1991--1999. MMWR Surveill Summ 2003; 52(2): 1-8.

[2] Wong JA, Clark JF. Correlation of symptoms with age and location of gestation in tubal pregnancy. *J. Natl. Med. Assoc.* 1968; 60(3): 221-3.

[3] Centers for Disease Control and Prevention (CDC). Ectopic pregnancy mortality - Florida, 2009-2010. *MMWR Morb. Mortal Wkly Rep* 2012; 61(6): 106-9.

[4] Capmas P, Bouyer J, Fernandez H. Treatment of ectopic pregnancies in 2014: new answers to some old questions. *Fertil. Steril.* 2014; 101(3): 615-20.

[5] Tait L. Five cases of extra-uterine pregnancy operated upon at the time of rupture. *Br. Med. J.* 1884; 1(1226): 1250-1.

[6] Lund J. Early ectopic pregnancy; comments on conservative treatment. *J. Obstet. Gynaecol.* Br. Emp. 1955; 62(1): 70-6.

[7] Mashiach S, Carp HJ, Serr DM. Nonoperative management of ectopic pregnancy. A preliminary report. *J. Reprod. Med.* 1982; 27(3): 127-32.

[8] Craig LB, Khan S. Expectant management of ectopic pregnancy. Clin. *Obstet. Gynecol.* 2012; 55(2): 461-70.

[9] Korhonen J, Stenman UH, Ylöstalo P. Low-dose oral methotrexate with expectant management of ectopic pregnancy. *Obstet. Gynecol.* 1996; 88(5): 775-8.

[10] Egarter C, Kiss H, Husslein P. Prostaglandin versus expectant management in early tubal pregnancy. *Prostaglandins Leukot Essent Fatty Acids* 1991; 42(3): 177-9.

[11] Hajenius PJ, Mol F, Mol BW, Bossuyt PM, Ankum WM, van der Veen F. Interventions for tubal ectopic pregnancy. *Cochrane Database Syst. Rev.* 2007 Jan 24; (1): CD000324.

[12] van Mello NM, Mol F, Verhoeve HR, van Wely M, Adriaanse AH, Boss EA, Dijkman AB, Bayram N, Emanuel MH, Friederich J, van der Leeuw-Harmsen L, Lips JP, Van Kessel MA, Ankum WM, van der Veen F, Mol BW, Hajenius PJ. Methotrexate or expectant management in women with an ectopic pregnancy or pregnancy of unknown location and low serum hCG concentrations? A randomized comparison. *Hum. Reprod.* 2013; 28(1): 60-7.

[13] Ylöstalo P, Cacciatore B, Sjöberg J, Kääriäinen M, Tenhunen A, Stenman UH. Expectant management of ectopic pregnancy. *Obstet. Gynecol.* 1992; 80(3 Pt 1): 345-8.

[14] Mavrelos D, Nicks H, Jamil A, Hoo W, Jauniaux E, Jurkovic D. Efficacy and safety of a clinical protocol for expectant management of selected women diagnosed with a tubal ectopic pregnancy. *Ultrasound Obstet. Gynecol.* 2013; 42(1): 102-7.

[15] Buster JE, Krotz S. Reproductive performance after ectopic pregnancy. *Semin. Reprod. Med.* 2007; 25(2): 131-3.

[16] Helmy S, Sawyer E, Ofili-Yebovi D, Yazbek J, Ben Nagi J, Jurkovic D. Fertility outcomes following expectant management of tubal ectopic pregnancy. *Ultrasound Obstet. Gynecol.* 2007; 30(7): 988-93.

[17] Juneau C, Bates GW. Reproductive outcomes after medical and surgical management of ectopic pregnancy. *Clin. Obstet. Gynecol.* 2012; 55(2): 455-60.

[18] Stika CS. Methotrexate: the pharmacology behind medical treatment for ectopic pregnancy. *Clin. Obstet. Gynecol.* 2012; 55(2): 433-9.

[19] Tanaka T, Hayashi H, Kutsuzawa T, Fujimoto S, Ichinoe K. Treatment of interstitial ectopic pregnancy with methotrexate: report of a successful case. *Fertil. Steril.* 1982; 37(6): 851-2.

[20] Ory SJ, Villanueva AL, Sand PK, Tamura RK. Conservative treatment of ectopic pregnancy with methotrexate. *Am. J. Obstet. Gynecol.* 1986; 154(6): 1299-306.

[21] Stovall TG, Ling FW, Buster JE. Outpatient chemotherapy of unruptured ectopic pregnancy. *Fertil. Steril.* 1989; 51(3): 435-8.

[22] Stovall TG, Ling FW. Single-dose methotrexate: an expanded clinical trial. *Am. J. Obstet. Gynecol.* 1993; 168(6 Pt 1): 1759-62; discussion 1762-5.

[23] Morlock RJ, Lafata JE, Eisenstein D. Cost-effectiveness of single-dose methotrexate compared with laparoscopic treatment of ectopic pregnancy. *Obstet. Gynecol.* 2000; 95(3): 407-12.

[24] Fernandez H, Lelaidier C, Thouvenez V, Frydman R. The use of a pretherapeutic, predictive score to determine inclusion criteria for the non-surgical treatment of ectopic pregnancy. *Hum. Reprod.* 1991; 6(7): 995-8.

[25] Pfeifer S, Goldberg J, Lobo R, Thomas M, Widra E, Licht M, et al. Medical treatment of ectopic pregnancy: a committee opinion. Practice Committee of American Society for Reproductive Medicine. *Fertil. Steril.* 2013; 100(3): 638-44.

[26] Bachman EA, Barnhart K. Medical management of ectopic pregnancy: a comparison of regimens. *Clin. Obstet. Gynecol.* 2012; 55(2): 440-7.

[27] Goldstein DP, Goldstein PR, Bottomley P, Osathanondh R, Marean AR. Methotrexate with citrovorum factor rescue for nonmetastatic gestational trophoblastic neoplasms. *Obstet. Gynecol.* 1976; 48(3): 321-3.

[28] Bagshawe KD, Dent J, Newlands ES, Begent RH, Rustin GJ. The role of low-dose methotrexate and folinic acid in gestational trophoblastic tumours (GTT). *Br. J. Obstet. Gynaecol.* 1989; 96(7): 795-802.

[29] Barnhart KT, Gosman G, Ashby R, Sammel M. The medical management of ectopic pregnancy: a meta-analysis comparing "single dose" and "multidose" regimens. *Obstet. Gynecol.* 2003; 101(4): 778-84.

[30] Lipscomb GH, Meyer NL, Flynn DE, Peterson M, Ling FW. Oral methotrexate for treatment of ectopic pregnancy. *Am. J. Obstet. Gynecol.* 2002; 186(6): 1192-5.

[31] Jamal HS, Amarin Z. Laparoscopic methotrexate instillation in unruptured tubal pregnancy--is it worthwhile? *J. Obstet. Gynaecol.* 2001; 21(4): 402-4.

[32] Gervaise A, Fernandez H. Methotrexate administration in the treatment of unruptured tubal pregnancy. Prospective non-randomized study: intramuscular injection versus transvaginal sonography-guided injection. *J. Gynecol. Obstet. Biol. Reprod.* (Paris) 2003; 32(5): 420-5.

[33] Goldenberg M, Bider D, Oelsner G, Admon D, Mashiach S. Treatment of interstitial pregnancy with methotrexate via hysteroscopy. *Fertil. Steril.* 1992; 58(6): 1234-6.

[34] Levin I, Tsafrir Z, Sa' ar N, Lessing J, Avni A, Gamzu R, Almog B. "Watchful waiting" in ectopic pregnancies: a balance between reduced success rates and less methotrexate. *Fertil. Steril.* 2011; 95(3): 1159-60.

[35] Cohen A, Zakar L, Gil Y, Amer-Alshiek J, Bibi G, Almog B, Levin I. Methotrexate success rates in progressing ectopic pregnancies: a reappraisal. *Am. J. Obstet. Gynecol.* 2014 Mar 19. pii: S0002-9378(14)00271-3. doi: 10.1016/j.ajog.2014.03.043.

[36] de Bennetot M, Rabischong B, Aublet-Cuvelier B, Belard F, Fernandez H, Bouyer J, Canis M, Pouly JL. Fertility after tubal ectopic pregnancy: results of a population-based study. *Fertil. Steril.* 2012; 98(5): 1271-6.e1-3.

[37] Allonier C, Ego A, Gerbaud L, Job-Spira N, Subtil D, Bouyer J. Comparison of fertility rates after ectopic pregnancy in Auvergne and Lille regions. *J. Gynecol. Obstet. Biol. Reprod.* (Paris) 2003; 32(5): 439-46.

[38] Bouyer J, Fernandez H, Coste J, Pouly JL, Job-Spira N. Fertility after ectopic pregnancy: 10-year results in the Auvergne Registry. *J. Gynecol. Obstet. Biol. Repro*d. (Paris) 2003; 32(5): 431-8.

[39] Fernandez H, Yves Vincent SC, Pauthier S, Audibert F, Frydman R. Randomized trial of conservative laparoscopic treatment and methotrexate administration in ectopic pregnancy and subsequent fertility. *Hum. Reprod.* 1998; 13(11): 3239-43.

[40] Dias Pereira G, Hajenius PJ, Mol BW, Ankum WM, Hemrika DJ, Bossuyt PM, van der Veen F. Fertility outcome after systemic methotrexate and laparoscopic salpingostomy for tubal pregnancy. *Lancet* 1999; 353(9154): 724-5.

[41] Fernandez H, Capmas P, Lucot JP, Resch B, Panel P, Bouyer J; GROG. Fertility after ectopic pregnancy: the DEMETER randomized trial. *Hum. Reprod.* 2013; 28(5): 1247-53.

[42] Boots CE, Gustofson RL, Feinberg EC. Does methotrexate administration for ectopic pregnancy after in vitro fertilization impact ovarian reserve or ovarian responsiveness? *Fertil. Steril.* 2013; 100(6): 1590-3.

[43] Orvieto R, Kruchkovich J, Zohav E, Rabinson J, Anteby EY, Meltcer S. Does methotrexate treatment for ectopic pregnancy influence the patient's performance during a subsequent in vitro fertilization/embryo transfer cycle? *Fertil. Steril.* 2007; 88(6): 1685-6.

[44] Oriol B, Barrio A, Pacheco A, Serna J, Zuzuarregui JL, Garcia-Velasco JA. Systemic methotrexate to treat ectopic pregnancy does not affect ovarian reserve. *Fertil. Steril.* 2008; 90(5): 1579-82.

[45] Provansal M, Agostini A, Lacroix O, Gerbeau S, Grillo JM, Gamerre M. Ultrasound monitoring in patients undergoing in-vitro fertilization after methotrexate treatment for ectopic pregnancy. *Ultrasound Obstet. Gynecol.* 2009; 34(6): 715-9.

[46] McLaren JF, Burney RO, Milki AA, Westphal LM, Dahan MH, Lathi RB. Effect of methotrexate exposure on subsequent fertility in women undergoing controlled ovarian stimulation. *Fertil. Steril.* 2009; 92(2): 515-9.

[47] Saraj AJ, Wilcox JG, Najmabadi S, Stein SM, Johnson MB, Paulson RJ. Resolution of hormonal markers of ectopic gestation: a randomized trial comparing single-dose intramuscular methotrexate with salpingostomy. *Obstet. Gynecol.* 1998; 92(6): 989-94.

[48] Sowter MC, Farquhar CM, Petrie KJ, Gudex G. A randomised trial comparing single dose systemic methotrexate and laparoscopic surgery for the treatment of unruptured tubal pregnancy. *BJOG* 2001; 108(2): 192-203.

[49] Colacurci N, De Franciscis P, Zarcone R, Fortunato N, Passaro M, Mollo A, Russo G. Time length of negativization of hCG serum values after either surgical or medical treatment of ectopic pregnancy. *Panminerva Med.* 1998; 40(3): 223-5.

[50] Sowter MC, Farquhar CM, Gudex G. An economic evaluation of single dose systemic methotrexate and laparoscopic surgery for the treatment of unruptured ectopic pregnancy. *BJOG* 2001; 108(2): 204-12.

[51] Nieuwkerk PT, Hajenius PJ, Ankum WM, Van der Veen F, Wijker W, Bossuyt PM. Systemic methotrexate therapy versus laparoscopic salpingostomy in patients with tubal pregnancy. Part I. Impact on patients' health-related quality of life. *Fertil. Steril.* 1998; 70(3): 511-7.

[52] Nieuwkerk PT, Hajenius PJ, Van der Veen F, Ankum WM, Wijker W, Bossuyt PM. Systemic methotrexate therapy versus laparoscopic salpingostomy in tubal pregnancy. Part II. Patient preferences for systemic methotrexate. *Fertil. Steril.* 1998; 70(3): 518-22.

[53] Deepa J, Oladimeji O, Funlayo O. Factors that determine patient satisfaction after surgical treatment of ectopic pregnancy: improving the patient journey. *Eur. J. Obstet. Gynecol. Reprod. Biol.* 2014; 178: 60-5.

[54] Hsu S, Mitwally MF, Aly A, Al-Saleh M, Batt RE, Yeh J. Laparoscopic management of tubal ectopic pregnancy in obese women. *Fertil. Steril.* 2004; 81(1): 198-202.

[55] Tulandi T, Kabli N. Laparoscopy in patients with bleeding ectopic pregnancy. *J. Obstet. Gynaecol. Can.* 2006; 28(5): 361-5.

[56] Byron JW, Markenson G, Miyazawa K. A randomized comparison of Verres needle and direct trocar insertion for laparoscopy. *Surg. Gynecol. Obstet.* 1993; 177(3): 259-62.

[57] Bruhat MA, Manhes H, Mage G, Pouly JL. Treatment of ectopic pregnancy by means of laparoscopy. *Fertil. Steril.* 1980; 33(4): 411-4.

[58] Tulandi T, Guralnick M. Treatment of tubal ectopic pregnancy by salpingotomy with or without tubal suturing and salpingectomy. *Fertil. Steril.* 1991; 55(1): 53-5.

[59] Stock L, Milad M. Surgical management of ectopic pregnancy. *Clin. Obstet. Gynecol.* 2012; 55 (2): 448-54.

[60] Maymon R, Shulman A, Halperin R, Michell A, Bukovsky I. Ectopic pregnancy and laparoscopy: review of 1197 patients treated by salpingectomy or salpingotomy. *Eur. J. Obstet. Gynecol. Reprod. Biol.* 1995; 62(1): 61-7.

[61] Kelly RW, Martin SA, Strickler RC. Delayed hemorrhage in conservative surgery for ectopic pregnancy. *Am. J. Obstet. Gynecol.* 1979; 133(2): 225-6.

[62] Mol F, van Mello NM, Strandell A, Strandell K, Jurkovic D, Ross J, et al. Salpingotomy versus salpingectomy in women with tubal pregnancy (ESEP study): an open-label, multicentre, randomised controlled trial. *Lancet* 2014; 383(9927): 1483-9.

[63] Kayatas S, Demirci O, Kumru P, Mahmutoglu D, Saribrahim B, Arinkan SA. Predictive factors for failure of salpingostomy in ectopic pregnancy. *J. Obstet. Gynaecol. Res.* 2014; 40(2): 453-8.

[64] Milad MP, Klein E, Kazer RR. Preoperative serum hCG level and intraoperative failure of laparoscopic linear salpingostomy for ectopic pregnancy. *Obstet. Gynecol.* 1998; 92(3): 373-6.

[65] Graczykowski JW, Mishell DR Jr. Methotrexate prophylaxis for persistent ectopic pregnancy after conservative treatment by salpingostomy. *Obstet. Gynecol.* 1997; 89(1): 118-22.

[66] Pouly JL, Chapron C, Canis M, Mage G, Wattiez A, Manhes H, Bruhat MA. Subsequent fertility for patients presenting with an ectopic pregnancy and having an intra-uterine device in situ. *Hum. Reprod.* 1991; 6(7): 999-1001.

[67] Clausen I. Conservative versus radical surgery for tubal pregnancy. A review. *Acta. Obstet. Gynecol. Scand.* 1996; 75: 8–12.

[68] Silva PD, Schaper AM, Rooney B. Reproductive outcome after 143 laparoscopic procedures for ectopic pregnancy. *Obstet. Gynecol.* 1993; 81: 710–5.

[69] Dubuisson JB, Aubriot FX, Foulot H, Bruel D, Bouquet de la Jolini_ere J, Mandelbrot L. Reproductive outcome after laparoscopic salpingectomy for tubal pregnancy. *Fertil. Steril.* 1990; 53: 1004–7.

[70] Yao M, Tulandi T. Current status of surgical and nonsurgical management of ectopic pregnancy. *Fertil. Steril.* 1997; 67: 421–33.

[71] Mol BW, Matthijsse HC, Tinga DJ, Huynh T, Hajenius PJ, Ankum WM, et al. Fertility after conservative and radical surgery for tubal pregnancy. *Hum. Reprod.* 1998; 13: 1804–9.

[72] Bangsgaard N, Lund CO, Ottesen B, Nilas L. Improved fertility following conservative surgical treatment of ectopic pregnancy. *BJOG* 2003; 110: 765–70.

[73] Mol F, van Mello NM, Strandell A, Strandell K, Jurkovic D, Ross J et al. Salpingotomy versus salpingectomy in women with tubal pregnancy (ESEP study): an open-label, multicentre, randomised controlled trial. *Lancet* 2014; 383(9927): 1483-9.

[74] D'Hooghe T, Tomassetti C. Surgery for ectopic pregnancy: making the right choice. *Lancet* 2014; 383(9927): 1444-5.

[75] Dubuisson JB, Aubriot FX, Cardone V. Laparoscopic salpingectomy for tubal pregnancy. *Fertil. Steril.* 1987; 47(2): 225-8.

[76] Damario M, Rock J. Ectopic pregnancy. In: Rock J, Jones H, eds. Te Linde's Operative Gynecology. Philadelphia: Wolters Kluwer/Lippincott Williams and Wilkins; 2008: 798–824.

[77] Kim YW, Park BJ, Kim TE, Ro DY. Single-port laparoscopic salpingectomy for surgical treatment of tubal pregnancy: comparison with multi-port laparoscopic salpingectomy. *Int. J. Med. Sci.* 2013; 10(8): 1073-8

[78] Jurkovic D, Wilkinson H. Diagnosis and management of ectopic pregnancy. BMJ 2011 Jun 10; 342: d3397. doi: 10.1136/bmj.d3397.

[79] Wang LL, Xi QK. Application and study of miphasiton at home and abroad. *J. Practical. Obstet. Gynecol.* 1997; 13: 72-73.

[80] Gazvani MR, Baruah DN, Alfirevic Z, Emery SJ. Mifepristone in combination with methotrexate for the medical treatment of tubal pregnancy: a randomized, controlled trial. *Hum. Reprod.* 1998; 13: 1987-90.

[81] Perdu M, Camus E, Rozenberg P, Goffinet F, Chastang C, Philippe HJ, Nisand I. Treating ectopic pregnancy with the combination of mifepristone and methotrexate: a phase II nonrandomized study. *Am. J. Obstet. Gynecol.* 1998; 179: 640-3.

[82] Lozeau AM, Potter B. Diagnosis and management of ectopic pregnancy. *Am. Fam. Physician* 2005; 72: 1707-14.

[83] Rozenberg P, Chevret S, Camus E, de Tayrac R, Garbin O, de Poncheville L et al. Medical treatment of ectopic pregnancies: a randomized clinical trial comparing methotrexate-mifepristone and methotrexate-placebo. *Hum. Reprod.* 2003; 18: 1802-8.

[84] Ransom MX, Garcia AJ, Bohrer M, Corsan GH, Kemmann E. Serum progesterone as a predictor of methotrexate success in the treatment of ectopic pregnancy. *Obstet. Gynecol.* 1994; 83: 1033-7.

[85] Corsan GH, Karacan M, Qasim S, Bohrer MK, Ransom MX, Kemmann E. Identification of hormonal parameters for successful systemic single-dose methotrexate therapy in ectopic pregnancy. *Hum. Reprod.* 1995; 10: 2719-22.

[86] Paris FX, Henry-Suchet J, Tesquier L, Dacquin G, Pez JP, Loysel T, Loffredo V, Roger M, De Brux J. Effect of an antiprogesterone (RU 486) on extra-uterine pregnancy. *Rev. Fr. Gynecol. Obstet.* 1986; 81: 607-9.

[87] Labeling changes for mifepristone. *FDA Consum* 2005 Jan-Feb; 39 (1): 5.

[88] Grossman N. Use of mifepristone for treatment of ectopic pregnancy. *Am. Fam. Physician* 2006; 73: 1703.

[89] Nilsson UW, Johns TG, Wilmann T, Kaitu' u-Lino T, Whitehead C, Dimitriadis E, Menkhorst E, Saglam B, Gao Y, Greenall SA, Horne AW, Tong S. Effects of gefitinib, an epidermal growth factor receptor inhibitor, on human placental cell growth. *Obstet. Gynecol.* 2013; 122(4): 737-44.

[90] Skubisz MM, Horne AW, Johns TG, Nilsson UW, Duncan WC, Wallace EM, Critchley HO, Tong S. Combination gefitinib and methotrexate compared with methotrexate alone to treat ectopic pregnancy. *Obstet. Gynecol.* 2013; 122(4): 745-51.

[91] Horne AW, Skubisz MM, Doust A, Duncan WC, Wallace E, Critchley HO, Johns TG, Norman JE, Bhattacharya S, Mollison J, Rassmusen M, Tong S. Phase II single arm open label multicentre clinical trial to evaluate the efficacy and side effects of a combination of gefitinib and methotrexate to treat tubal ectopic pregnancies (GEM II): study protocol.

BMJ Open 2013 Jul 19; 3(7). pii: e002902. doi: 10.1136/bmjopen-2013-002902.

[92] Sowter MC, Farquhar CM. Ectopic pregnancy: an update. Curr. Opin. Obstet. Gynecol. 2004; 16: 289-93.

[93] Garbin O, de Tayrac R, de Poncheville L, Coiffic J, Lucot JP, Le Goueff F, et al. Medical treatment of ectopic pregnancy: a randomized clinical trial comparing methotrexate-mifepristone and methotrexate-placebo. *J. Gynecol. Obstet. Biol. Reprod.* (Paris) 2004; 33: 391-400.

[94] Li ZH, Quan S. Mifepristone combined with methotrexate for conservative treatment of tubal ectopic pregnancy. *Di Yi Jun Yi Da Xue Xue Bao* 2004; 24: 829-31.

[95] Song HD, Chen SL, He JX, Qiu YW. Combined use of methotrexate and mifepristone for ectopic pregnancy management: a meta- analysis. *Nan Fang Yi Ke Da Xue Xue Bao* 2006; 26: 1815-7.

[96] Veena P. Use of mifepristone along with methotrexate in medical management of unruptured ectopic pregnancy. *J. Obstet. Gynaecol.* 2011; 31: 667. doi: 10.3109/01443615.2011.593651.

[97] Varma R, Gupta J. Tubal ectopic pregnancy. *Clin. Evid.* (Online) 2012; 10: 2012. pii: 1406.

In: Ectopic Pregnancy
Editor: Mallory T. Church

ISBN: 978-1-63463-260-7

Chapter 3

Ectopic Pregnancy: Old and New Insights in the Management

Elisa Picardo, Marco Mitidieri, Emilie Marion Canuto, Elena Minniti, Gianluigi Marchino, Chiara Benedetto and Saverio Danese
A.O.U. Città della Salute e della Scienza, Sant'Anna Hospital, Dipartimento di Ginecologia e Ostetricia, Torino, Italy

Abstract

In the developed world, the rate of ectopic pregnancies has been increasing up to 2% of all pregnancies in the last thirty years. The incidence is thought to be higher in developing countries, but specific numbers are unknown.

The majority of the ectopic pregnancies involve the fallopian tube (95%), followed by ovarian site (3.2%), abdominal site (1.3%), cervical site (0.15%), and cesarean scar site. Even if in the last two decades a lot have been written about this topic, its therapeutic management still raises concerns, and, at the present moment, no guidelines exist to help choosing the best treatment [1].

Diagnosis: Diagnosis of ectopic pregnancy has improved significantly thanks to the advances in ultrasound technology, rapid and sensitive serum hormone assays and an increased understanding of the associated risk factors. Despite this, the diagnosis remains difficult, and an ectopic pregnancy could still be missed: this happens to 12% - 45% of them at their first admission to emergency department [1]. That is why ectopic pregnancy remains the leading cause of death during the early trimester of pregnancy. Early diagnosis reduces the risk of tubal rupture and allows more conservative medical treatments to be employed, thus preserving subsequent fertility.

Management: Ectopic pregnancy may be managed expectantly, medically and surgically. In these days of increasing outpatient diagnosis and management it is important to remember the risks of ruptured ectopic pregnancy. Clear documentation of diagnostic and management strategies – with clinical, sonographic and biochemical assessment of the patient – is therefore important. Management is tailored to individual patients, always keeping in mind that women's preferences also depend on the way the treatment options are presented by the physician.

The activity of the ectopic pregnancy is pivotal in guiding treatment's choice. A very active ectopic pregnancy (hemodynamic failure, symptoms of rupture, high HCG) has a high risk of tubal rupture or has already ruptured and needs compulsorily a surgical treatment. For very inactive ectopic pregnancies (HCG < 1500 IU/L, plateau levels, asymptomatic woman) the best management could be a watchful wait, i.e., an intensive follow up until HCG normalization. However, in the other cases, the criteria for defining the activity of an ectopic pregnancy (i.e., pain, time of amenorrhea, hCG and progesterone level, size of hematosalpinx, and importance of hemoperitoneum, presence of a yolk sac, an embryo, or cardiac activity) and their cut off are still a matter of debate. Medical treatment is based on methotrexate, an antimetabolite, which is given at 1 mg/kg or 50 mg/m^2 according to different protocols, and has a reported success rate ranging from 63% to 96.7% [2,3]. Surgical treatment consists of conservative therapy or radical therapy: the first one has a 100% efficacy rate while the second one has a success rate ranging from 82.5% to 94.4% [4].

Subsequent fertility: Data about subsequent fertility are still to be confirmed: they all come from observational studies, conducted throughout a limited period, thus lacking adequate statistical power for definitive conclusions. Studies suggest that around 60% of women affected by an ectopic pregnancy go on to have a viable intra uterine pregnancy [4,5]. The comparison between medical treatment and surgical conservative treatment did not show statistically significant differences, and the same result comes when comparing conservative and radical surgery. The risk of recurrence is 5-20%, regardless of the treatment option chosen. However, the risk is reduced after each subsequent intrauterine pregnancy [5].

Bibliography

[1] Oron G, Tulandi T. A pragmatic and evidence-based management of ectopic pregnancy J Minim Invasive Gynecol. 2013 Jul-Aug;20[4]:446-54.
[2] Practice Committee of American Society for Reproductive Medicine et al. Medical treatment of ectopic pregnancy: a committee opinion. Fertil Steril. (2013)
[3] Alkatout I, Honemeyer U, Strauss A, et al. Clinical diagnosis and treatment of ectopic pregnancy Obstet Gynecol Surv. 2013 Aug;68[8]:571-81.
[4] Rana, P; Kazmi, I; Singh, R, et al. Ectopic pregnancy: a review Arch. Gynecol. Obstet., 2013 vol. 288[4] pp. 747-57.
[5] Capmas, P; Bouyer, J; Fernandez, H Treatment of ectopic pregnancies in 2014: new answers to some old questions Fertil. Steril., 2014 vol. 101[3] pp. 615-20.

Introduction

An ectopic pregnancy is a complication of pregnancy in which the blastocyst implants anywhere outside endometrial cavity of uterus. It is the major cause of maternal mortality during early pregnancy and accounts for 10% of all pregnancy- related deaths. Furthermore, it increases the chances of infertility as well as incidence of the subsequent ectopic pregnancy. In the developed world, the rate of ectopic pregnancies has been increasing up to 2% of all pregnancies in the last thirty years. The incidence is thought to be higher in developing countries, but specific numbers are unknown. The majority of the ectopic pregnancies involve the fallopian tube (95%), followed by ovarian site (3.2%), abdominal site (1.3%), cervical site (0.15%), and cesarean scar site (Table 1; Figure 1).

Even if in the last two decades a lot have been written about this topic, its therapeutic management still raises concerns, and, at the present moment, no guidelines exist to help choosing the best treatment.Early diagnosis reduces the risk of tubal rupture and allows more conservative medical treatments to be employed, thus preserving subsequent fertility. Diagnosis of ectopic pregnancy has improved significantly thanks to the advances in ultrasound technology, rapid and sensitive serum hormone assays and an increased understanding of the associated risk factors (as pelvic inflammatory disease, Chlamydia trachomatis infection, tubal surgery, induced conception cycle, endometriosis, previous ectopic pregnancy) Table 2. Despite this, the diagnosis remains difficult, and an ectopic pregnancy could still be missed: this happens to 12% - 45% of them at their first admission to emergency department [1, 2]. That is why ectopic pregnancy remains the leading cause of death during the early trimester of pregnancy.

Table 1. Different site for ectopic pregnancy

SITE	%
Tubal EP	90-95%
Cervical EP	0.15%
Ovarian EP	0.15%-3%
Caesarean scar EP	6%
Interstitial EP	2.5%
Abdominal EP	1.3%
Heterotopic EP	1-3%
Information from reference: Rana P., Kazmi I., Singh R., et al. Ectopic pregnancy: a review. Archives of gynecology and obstetrics, 288[4], 747-757.(2013)	

Table 2. Risk Factors for Ectopic Pregnancy

Risk factor	*Odds ratio (%) A higher odds ratio indicates a stronger risk factor*
Previous tubal surgery	21.0
Previous ectopic pregnancy	8.3
Previous genital infections	2.4 to 3.7
Infertility	2 to 2.5
Current smoking	2.3
Previous intrauterine device use	1.6
Information from references: - Ankum WM, Mol BW, Van der Veen F, Bossuyt PM. Risk factors for ectopic pregnancy: a meta-analysis. Fertil Steril 1996;65:1093-9. - Mol BW, Ankum WM, Bossuyt PM, Van der Veen F. Contraception and the risk of ectopic pregnancy: a meta-analysis. Contraception 1995;52:337-41.	

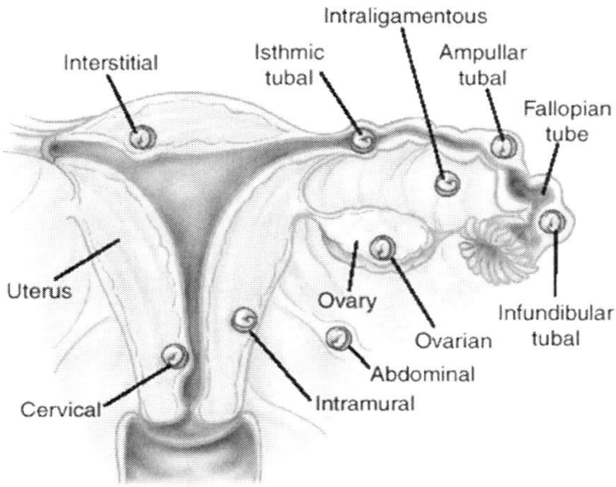

Figure1. Sites for Ectopic Pregnancy.

The differential diagnosis should consider other gynecological conditions and non gynecological conditions: in the former we include early stage of normal intrauterine pregnancy, abortion, torsion of ovary or fallopian tube, ovarian cyst, ruptured corpus luteum cyst or follicle, necrotic myoma, pelvic inflammatory disease and tubo-ovarian abscess; in the latter we include acute appendicitis, cystitis, pyelonephritis, nephrolithiasis, intra-abdominal inflammation Table 3.

The pillars of ectopic pregnancy diagnosis are three: symptoms, HCG serum levels pattern, transvaginal ultrasound. An ectopic pregnancy should be suspected in all patients in reproductive age presenting with amenorrhea of 6 to 8 weeks, nausea/vomiting, lower abdominal pain, abnormal uterine bleeding [3, 4]. Gynecologic examination can find an enlarged soft uterus, a painful adnexal mass, pelvic tenderness, and even peritoneal signs. HCG in a normal pregnancy doubles approximately every 1.5 days for the first 5 weeks of gestation and then every 3.5 days [5]. Ectopic pregnancy shows generally an abnormal pattern of HCG: it increases slowly and then reaches a plateau, or it decreases. Transvaginal ultrasound can detect an intrauterine chorionic sac starting from HCG levels of 1500- 2500 mIU/ml, also known as discriminatory zone: its absence thus implies an abnormal gestation [6-8]. In a normal intrauterine pregnancy a chorionic sac is observable, at 4.5 – 5 weeks of gestation, as a double echogenic ring around a hypoechoic gestational sac with eccentric embedding in the decidua [9, 10]. However, in some ectopic pregnancy, it is possible to detect a pseudosac in the uterine cavity: it is a blood collection surrounded by thick endometrium [11]. It is also important to keep in mind the possibility, even if really rare, of a heterotopic pregnancy, whose total number is rising due to the increase of assisted reproduction. Color Doppler and Power Doppler can show randomly dispersed multiple small vessels within the adnexa in presence of ectopic pregnancy [9, 10]. In case ultrasound does not give definitive diagnosis, HCG should be repeated every three days. Combining ecography and serial HCG levels allows reaching a sensitivity of 96% and a specificity of 97% in diagnosing an ectopic pregnancy.

Table 3. Differential Diagnosis of Ectopic Pregnancy

Differential Diagnosis of Ectopic Pregnancy	
Gynecological conditions	Non gynecological conditions
Normal intra uterine pregnancy - Miscarriage	Acute appendicitis
Tubo-ovarian abscess - Ovarian torsion	Cystitis
Ruptured corpus luteum cyst or follicle	Pyelonephritis
Pelvic inflammatory disease	Urinary calculi
Necrotic myoma	Intra-abdominal inflammation

Management

Ectopic pregnancy may be managed expectantly, medically, and surgically. The choice of treatment should first of all consider clinical conditions of the patient, but also patient's preference, after an appropriate counseling about monitoring, outcome, risks and benefits of each procedure.

The activity of the ectopic pregnancy is pivotal in guiding treatment's choice. The definition of activity is still a matter of debate [12]. A very active ectopic pregnancy presents with hemodynamic failure, symptoms of rupture such as pain and syncope, high HCG and has a high risk of tubal rupture or has already ruptured. This one needs compulsorily a surgical treatment. The surgical treatment could be conservative (salpingotomy) or radical (salpingectomy). They are generally performed laparoscopically. Salpingotomy consists of an incision over the bulging portion of the tube and removing the ectopic mass with a 10 mm irrigation probe for hydrodissection, then the tubal incision is left open to allow secondary healing, while the pelvis is irrigated [13]. Serial HCG measurements should be carried out once a week until undetectable, to be sure that ectopic pregnancy has been completely treated. The problems of the conservative technique are the risk of persistence of trophoblastic cells, with failure rates ranging from 6.6% to 17.5% [13-19] and the risk of recurrence. A randomized trial proposed a routine prophylactic postoperative injection of methotrexate, showing a statistically significant decrease of persistent trophoblasts: 17.5% vs 0 ($p > 0.05$) [20]; this also allowed a shorter duration of postoperative follow up [16]. The DEMETER trial, a multicenter prospective trial concerning the subsequent fertility for treated ectopic pregnancies, confirmed a lower rate of persistence of trophoblastic cells (0.6%) [21]. Salpingectomy implies the removal of the tube from the horn to the fimbrial portion through dissection of the mesosalpinx and the fallopian tube with bipolar electrocautery forceps and scissors. This procedure has a 100% efficacy rate. The choice between conservative and radical treatment must consider patient's preferences and patient's history, but is often made during laparoscopy, considering the contralateral tube and the possibility to achieve a good hemostasis. Surgical treatment consists of conservative therapy or radical therapy: the first one has a 100% efficacy rate while the second one has a success rate ranging from 82.5% to 94.4% .

For very inactive ectopic pregnancies (HCG < 1500 IU/L, plateauing or decreasing levels, asymptomatic woman) the best management could be a watchful wait, i.e., an intensive follow up until HCG normalization [22]. The METEX trial, a multicenter randomized trial on women with low and plateauing HCG levels, failed to demonstrate differences between expectant management and methotrexate [15]. The American College of Obstetricians and Gynecologists suggests expectant management only in limited clinical situations, when ectopic pregnancy is suspected but TV ultrasound does not show a gestational sac or an extrauterine mass suspicious for an ectopic pregnancy and BHCG is low (< 200 IU/L) and declining [23].

However, in the other cases, the criteria for defining the activity of an ectopic pregnancy (i.e., pain, time of amenorrhea, hCG and progesterone level, size of hematosalpinx, and importance of hemoperitoneum, presence of a yolk sac, an embryo, or cardiac activity) and their cut off are still a matter of debate. Fernandez has created a score based on pain measurement, time of amenorrhea, HCG and Progesterone level, size of hematosalpinx, hemoperitoneum importance (Table 4) [21]. Nowadays, the cut off for defining a less active, and thus medically treatable, pregnancy varies from 1500 to 5000 IU/L HCG levels, with a preference for the higher threshold [24-28]. Medical treatment is based on methotrexate, an antimetabolite that acts on actively proliferating cells, which is given at 1 mg/kg or 50 mg/m2 according to different protocols, and has a reported success rate ranging from 63% to 96.7%. The heterogeneity of this results depends on variations in patients characteristics, study inclusion criteria, pretreatment HCG levels, MTX protocols, and on the different definitions of treatment failure. The lower the HCG level at the beginning, the higher the success rate is [6]. Pre treatment monitoring includes evaluation of uterine cavity to exclude the possibility of a coexisting intrauterine pregnancy, blood sampling with complete blood count, renal and liver function tests, blood group.

Table 4. Fernandez's score

	1	2	3
Gestational age (since amenorrhoea)	>49 days	42– 49 days	<42 days
HCG (mUI/ml)	1000	1000– 5000	>5000
Progesterone (ng/ml)	5	5– 10	>10
Tubal haematoma	None	Provoked	Spontaneous
Haematosalpinx (mm)	10	10– 30	>30
Peritoneal fluid (ml)	0	1– 100	>100

Fernandez's score includes six items that reflect activity of EP. When the score is low (under 13), the EP is considered to be not very active and is less likely to cause a tubal rupture.

Modified from H. Fernandez, P. Capmas, J.P.Lucot, B.Resch, P.Panel and J.Bouyer1, for the GROG Fertility after ectopic pregnancy: the DEMETER randomized trial Human Reproduction, Vol.28, No.5 pp. 1247–1253, 2013.

The ideal candidate for medical treatment is a patient hemodinamically stable, asymptomatic, compliant to follow up, with normal baseline liver and renal function tests. Two regimens are possible: multidose MTX (mtx 1.0 mg/kg i.m. daily at days 1,3,5,and 7 alternated with folinic acid on days 2,4,6,and 8) or single dose MTX (MTX 50 mg/m2). Three randomized trials showed that single dose success rate is comparable with that of multidose regimen [29-31]. Multidose regimen could be more appropriate in case of non tubal pregnancies including interstitial or cervical pregnancies [32]. Time to resolution after methotrexate injection is 3 to 7 weeks. HCG level has to be checked at day 1, day 4 and day 7. If HCG levels do not decline to greater than 15% between day 4 and 7, a second dose has to be given, and this happens in

Table 5. Contraindications to Medical Management of Ectopic Pregnancy with Systemic Methotrexate*

Contraindication	ACOG†	ASRM‡
Absolute contraindications	Breast-feeding; laboratory evidence of immunodeficiency; preexisting blood dyscrasias (*bone marrow hypoplasia, leukopenia, thrombocytopenia, or clinically significant anemia*); known sensitivity to methotrexate; active pulmonary disease; peptic ulcer disease; hepatic, renal, or hematologic dysfunction; alcoholism; alcoholic or other chronic liver disease	Breast-feeding; evidence of immunodeficiency; moderate-to-severe anemia, leukopenia, or thrombocytopenia; sensitivity to methotrexate; active pulmonary or peptic ulcer disease; clinically important hepatic or renal dysfunction; intrauterine pregnancy
Relative contraindications	Ectopic mass >3.5 cm; embryonic cardiac motion	Ectopic mass >4 cm detected by transvaginal ultrasonography; embryonic cardiac activity detected by transvaginal ultrasonography; patient declines blood transfusion; patient is not able to participate in follow-up; high initial hCG level (>5000 mIU/ml)
Choice of regimen based on hCG level	Multidose regimen of methotrexate may be appropriate if presenting hCG value >5000 mIU/ml	Single-dose regimen of methotrexate better in patients with a low initial hCG level

* ACOG denotes American College of Obstetricians and Gynecologists, and ASRM American Society for Reproductive Medicine.

† Data are from the American College of Obstetricians and Gynecologists. (ACOG Practice Bulletin no. 94: medical management of ectopic pregnancy. Obstet Gynecol 2008;111:1479-85.)

‡ Data are from the Practice Committee of the American Society for Reproductive Medicine. (Practice Committee of the American Society for Reproductive Medicine. Medical treatment of ectopic pregnancy. Fertil Steril 2006;86:Suppl:S96-S102.)

Modified from Barnhart, Kurt T. "Ectopic pregnancy." New England Journal of Medicine 361.4 (2009): 379-387.

15-20% of patients [33, 34]. Then HCG has to be checked weekly and an ultrasound has to be performed until HCG is < 5 UI/L [40-45]. Predictors of MTX failure are high initial HCG levels, (above 5000 UI/L), gestational mass > 4cm, presence of free peritoneal blood, rapidly increasing HCG concentrations (> 50% in 48h) before MTX administration, continued HCG rise during MTX [35-39].

More frequent side effects of MTX are bone marrow suppression, aphthous stomatitis, conjunctivitis, elevation of liver enzymes, stomatitis, nausea, diarrhea, but they are generally moderate and self limiting [22] (Table 5).

In situ injection of methotrexate with sonographic guidance is often used for extratubal ectopic pregnancies [46–49] but may also be used for tubal pregnancies. The addition of folinic acid to methotrexate therapy has not been found to provide any advantages: the half-life of methotrexate is very short, and even with the four-injection protocol the methotrexate dose is very low compared with the levels used in rheumatology or oncology [50]. Hyperosmolar glucose has also been injected into the fallopian tube under sonographic guidance to resolve ectopic pregnancies. Although it has been replaced by methotrexate as a general rule, it is often still used in heterotopic pregnancies when the use of methotrexate is contraindicated [51–54].

Subsequent Fertility

Data about subsequent fertility are still to be confirmed: they all come from observational studies, conducted throughout a limited period, thus lacking adequate statistical power for definitive conclusions. Studies suggest that around 60% of women affected by an ectopic pregnancy go on to have a viable intra uterine pregnancy. The comparison between medical treatment and surgical conservative treatment did not show statistically significant differences, and the same result comes when comparing conservative and radical surgery. The risk of recurrence is 5-20%, regardless of the treatment option chosen. However, the risk is reduced after each subsequent intrauterine pregnancy.

Cervical Ectopic Pregnancy

Cervical pregnancy is a rare type of ectopic pregnancy in which the pregnancy implants in the lining of the endocervical canal. Its incidence is 1:16000 to 1:18000 of all pregnancies and 0.1% of all ectopic pregnancies (Figure 3) [55].

Cervical pregnancy is often associated with significant morbidity and devastating effects on future fertility.

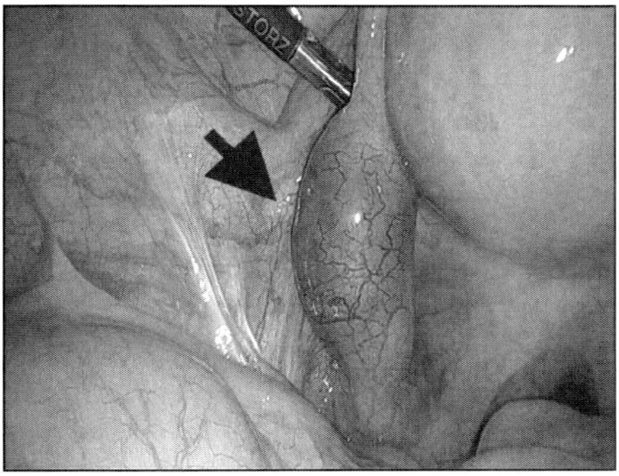

Figure 2. Tubaric Ectopic Pregnancy.

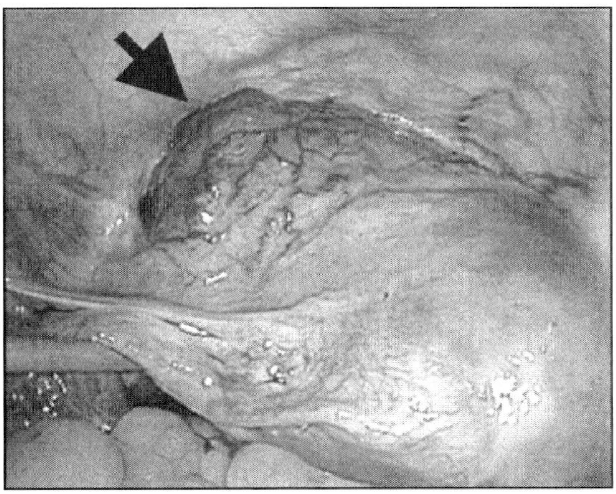

Figure 3. Cervical Ectopic Pregnancy.

This can be due to the deep penetrative effect of the trophoblast through the cervical walls and into the uterine blood supply. Historically, 70% of the reported cases required hysterectomy for massive blood loss [56]. The maternal mortality is reported to be 0% to 6% [57, 58].

The causes of cervical pregnancy remain unknown. The rarity of the condition has prevented any retrospective study with adequate numbers to determine the potential risk factors. Several studies have shown a high incidence of prior dilation and curettage among women with cervical pregnancies [59, 60], especially when the curettage damaged the endometrial lining and prevented implantation of the fertilized ovum. Endometrial inflammation from the use of an intrauterine device and pelvic inflammatory disease could also be a contributing factor [61]. Painless vaginal bleeding is the most common presentation, with only one third of women presenting by massive hemorrhage. In 1959, Paalman and McElin [62] offered 5 clinical signs to establish the diagnosis as follows:

1) uterine bleeding without cramping pain after a period of amenorrhea
2) softened and disproportionately enlarged cervix equal to or larger than the corporal portion of the uterus (an hourglass-shaped uterus)
3) products of conception entirely confined within, and firmly attached to, the endocervix
4) a snug internal os
5) a partially opened external os

The combination of transvaginal and transabdominal ultrasonography using high-resolution transducers would establish a diagnosis in most of the cases in the first trimester. This is essential because only cases diagnosed before 12 weeks, that is, before the trophoblast has infiltrated too deeply into the cervical wall, are amenable to conservative treatment.

In 1978, Raskin [63] suggested 4 sonographic diagnostic criteria as follows:

1) Enlargement of the cervix
2) Uterine enlargement
3) Diffuse amorphous intrauterine echoes
4) Absence of intrauterine pregnancy

There are other two diagnostic criteria in order to distinguish cervical ectopic pregnancy from an aborting intrauterine pregnancy residing in the cervix as follows [64]:

1) The "sliding sign" detected on transvaginal ultrasound examination, when the gestational sac of an abortus slides against the endocervial canal after gentle pressure on the cervix with the vaginal probe. This sign would not be seen in an implanted cervical pregnancy
2) The demonstration of peritrophoblastic blood flow to the conceptus by color flow Doppler ultrasonography. The nonviable sac, transiently passing through the cervix, will not have such blood flow and will show a positive sliding sign, and the closed internal os will differentiate it from an isthmicocervical pregnancy.

A sonographic impression of cervical pregnancy is correct in 87.5% of cases. However, when the ultrasound

is inconclusive, magnetic resonance imaging may be helpful in unusual or complicated cases [65].

Early detection is the key factor for conservative management. Methotrexate treatment of cervical pregnancy was first performed by Farabow et al. [66] in 1983.

The dose regimens of systemic methotrexate varied considerably. Single dose (50 mg/m2 intramuscularly [IM]) with monitoring of serum hCG levels on days 1,4 and 7 was described. If the difference in serum hCG levels is 15% or greater, the test is repeated weekly until it becomes undetectable. If the difference is less than 15%, methotrexate dose should be repeated, and new day 1 is begun. Multiple-dose regimens can also be used (1 mg/kg on days 1, 3, 5 and 7 IM), with or without 0.1 mg/kg of folinic acid rescue on alternate days. No more than 5 doses of methotrexate are to be given without a gap of 1 week. In 2009, an alternative high-dose regimen of methotrexate was suggested by Song et al. [67] in the form of a single course of 100 mg/m2 plus a dose of 200 mg/m2 in 500 mL of normal saline solution via intravenous injection with a 0.1 mg/kg of folinic acid rescue.

Methotrexate can also be used intracervically or intraamniotically in a dose of 50 mg/m2. However, there is a strong possibility of active bleeding after local injection, caused by rupture of the intra-amniotic membrane. Unfortunately, the present data are too limited and inconsistent to compare the efficacy of different regimens. The resolution time of cervical pregnancy after chemotherapy, as determined by serum hCG levels, varied from 2 to 5 weeks and, by sonographic appearance of the cervix, varied from 2 to 12 weeks. A possible problem with methotrexate therapy is the inability to predict the occurrence of massive bleeding, after trophoblast shedding, from the uninvoluted and atonic cervix.

Current literature review showed that 49% of viable cervical pregnancies have required an additional operative procedure to eradicate the aberrant trophoblastic tissue.

Local injection of potassium chloride (KCl) (3–5mL of 2 mEq/mL) under transvaginal ultrasound guidance is an alternative to methotrexate treatment. This method has been used as a primary therapy and in combination with systemic chemotherapy or after failed systemic methotrexate treatment, with 90% success rate [56]. Thus, KCl injection can be a viable option in the treatment of heterotopic cervical pregnancy without the need for local or systemic chemotherapy. However, there is still a possibility of major hemorrhage or infection of the implantation site, and further procedures may be required.

Use of prostaglandins in cervical pregnancies was reported by few authors. Dall et al. [68] reported its use, both systemically and intra-amniotically, in a 9-week cervical pregnancy, but despite simultaneous curettage, intractable hemorrhage necessitated an emergency hysterectomy. Spitzer et al. [69] subsequently described 3 cases of first-trimester cervical pregnancy that were successfully treated with curettage and local prostaglandin instillation (12.5–25 *m*g of sulprostone) Hysteroscopic management of cervical pregnancy with intrauterine irrigation with 3.5% hydrogen peroxide (H2O2) has been performed on 10 cases by Kim et al. [70] and was found to be a safe and effective alternative treatment. Hydrogen peroxide solution releases a large amount of free oxygen via catalysis, which is very abundant in embryos and the yolk sac and induces cell death because of oxygen toxicity.

Mifepristone acts as a competitive antagonist to progesterone at the receptor level. It indirectly induces decidual breakdown, leading to trophoblast detachment and decreased syncytiotrophoblast production of hCG, which, in turn, causes decreased production of progesterone by the corpus luteum [71] The combination of mifepristone with methotrexate is claimed to prevent the development of embryos and speed up embryonic death, which would shorten the treatment time. The dose of mifepristone used was usually 25 to 75 mg twice daily for 3 to 5 days orally.

Intracervical or systemic injections of syntocinon and/or ergometrine have no role in the management of cervical pregnancy because the uterine cervix consists mainly of fibrous connective tissue with only 10% smooth muscle. However, they may have a role in cases of cervicoisthmic implantation because the isthmus area has 50% to 60% muscular connective elements.

Dilation and Curettage (Surgical Evacuation) alone carries a 40% risk for hysterectomy [72]. Attempts to evacuate the uterus digitally or instrumentally will produce violent hemorrhage, necessitating hysterectomy in most cases. If tamponade provides successful hemostasis primarily, severe secondary hemorrhage necessitating hysterectomy may, nevertheless, occur up to 6 weeks later.

The outcome is significantly better when combined with other medical or surgical methods to control blood loss and to prevent residual gestational tissue from active regrowth with the establishment of collateral circulation after uterine artery embolization (UAE).

Angiographic Embolization. Securing the blood supply to cervical pregnancy by angiographic UAE was first introduced in 1990 by Lobel et al. [73]. Gelfoam particles (Upjohn) or polyvinyl alcohol (Boston Scientific) provides temporary occlusion of the vessel for 2 to 6 weeks. Its advantages over other treatment modalities include shorter hospital stay, fewer laboratory follow-ups, fewer outpatient checkups, and prevention of hemorrhage. However, women should be appropriately counseled about the possible impairment of fertility, loss of ovarian reserve, and the occurrence of obstetric complications in future pregnancies. The risk factors of recurrent vaginal bleeding after UAE are fetal cardiac activity before therapy, persistent high hCG level, and recurrent flow signal around the intracervical gestational sac. In 2004, Kung et al. [74] used an alternative combination of laparoscopically assisted uterine artery ligation followed by hysteroscopic endocervical resection to successfully treat 6 cervical pregnancies.

Total abdominal hysterectomy is the treatment of choice for patients with cervical pregnancies diagnosed during the second trimester, with unstable vital signs and excessive vaginal bleeding, with associated uterine pathology, who are Jehovah's witnesses, and who have completed their families. However, there will still be an increased risk for urinary tract injury because of the enlarged barrel-shaped cervix.

The impact of cervical pregnancy on future fertility is largely unknown because of the rarity of the condition and the infrequency with which women were observed after treatment. It is also unclear whether there is an increased risk for recurrence. Women, therefore, should be counseled about the risk for future ectopic pregnancies, second-trimester pregnancy losses, and the potential need for subsequent prophylactic cervical cerclage.

In a review of 120 published cases of cervical pregnancy Ushakov et al. [57] found 37 pregnancies identified after conservative management of cervical pregnancy, 34 intrauterine pregnancies, 2 tubal pregnancies, and 1 repeat cervical pregnancy. Current literature review found 38 pregnancies identified after conservative management of cervical pregnancy; all of them were intrauterine pregnancies; 6 women had first-trimester spontaneous miscarriage, with subsequent full-term pregnancy in 3 of them; 1woman had surgical termination of pregnancy; 1 woman had preterm labor; 1 woman had intrauterine fetal death at 26 weeks; another one had 8 weeks of intrauterine pregnancy with unknown outcome; and 28 had successful pregnancy outcome at full term.

Interstitial Ectopic Pregnancy

Interstitial ectopic pregnancies develop in the uterine portion of the fallopian tube and account for 2–4% of all ectopic pregnancies (Figure 4).

In general, interstitial pregnancies become symptomatic later than the usual tubal pregnancies and hence tend to be diagnosed later. Should rupture of the uterus occur, hemorrhage may be profound. Rupture may occur in up to 20% of women who progress beyond 12 weeks' gestation [75]. The reported maternal mortality rate for interstitial pregnancy is as high as 2.5% [76, 77]. Traditionally, interstitial pregnancies were managed with laparotomy and cornual resection [76]. This may adversely affect subsequent pregnancies, with uterine rupture being a major concern [78, 79]. The availability of high resolution transvaginal ultrasound along with monitoring of human chorionic gonadotropin (hCG) levels, allows early diagnosis of interstitial pregnancy before rupture occurs, leaving an option for conservative treatment modalities. These include ultrasound-guided local injection of potassium chloride into the gestational sac [79], various laparoscopic procedures [80] or medical treatment with methotrexate (MTX), either injected locally into the gestational sac [10] or by systemic intramuscular injection, using single or multiple dose protocols [81]. Hysteroscopic removal of a cornual pregnancy has also been reported [82]. Data regarding future fertility and pregnancy outcomes for interstitial pregnancy are limited.

The traditional surgical management of interstitial pregnancy used to be laparotomy, or cornual resection for those who wanted to preserve their fertility. This may still be required when there is excessive hemoperitoneum and the typical delayed diagnosis.

The rapid evolution of transvaginal ultrasound together with the availability of sensitive hCG assays allow early detection of all types of ectopic pregnancies. With that, most interstitial pregnancies can be diagnosed before rupture occurs, leaving the option for conservative medical or surgical treatment. Although sonographic criteria for interstitial pregnancy were proposed by various authors [83], misdiagnosis is not uncommon, and may be as high as 42% [84]. MTX is the most extensively studied and used agent for medical treatment for unruptured extrauterine pregnancy. It was also used for the treatment of unruptured interstitial pregnancies with success rates between 86 and 94% [85]. Today, laparoscopy is the standard surgical management of ectopic and interstitial pregnancies in hemodynamically stable patients.

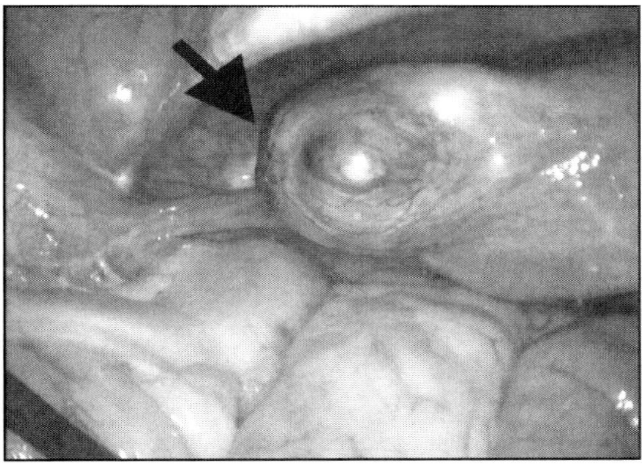

Figure 4. Interstitial Ectopic Pregnancy.

The first report on laparoscopic treatment of interstitial pregnancy was published by Reich et al. in 1988 [86]. Since then, others have reported on their experience and described conservative surgical techniques to allow preservation of future fertility and minimize the risk of uterine rupture in subsequent gestation. These conservative methods included the use of ligatures with or without local injection of vasopressin, or the encircling suture method prior to the removal of the gestational tissue. Laparoscopic surgery can be used even if hemodynamically unstable [87]. Few data exist regarding reproductive outcomes after treatment of interstitial pregnancy but another case series suggested that 75% succeeded in conceiving with an intrauterine pregnancy following treatment [81]. Although the exact risk of uterine rupture in subsequent pregnancy is unknown, women should be counseled carefully about this possibility.

Cesarean Scar Pregnancy

Cesarean scar pregnancy is a rare form of ectopic pregnancy, and its incidence may have been increased because of the increased rate of Cesarean sections performed (Figure 5). The incidence of Cesarean scar pregnancy was 1 : 2216. The exact cause of Cesarean scar pregnancy is still unknown. Nonetheless, its occurrence may be linked to an existing scar defect or microscopic dehiscent tract generated between the prior Cesarean scar and the endometrial canal [88]. Such tracts or wedge defects, likely resulting from previous Cesarean sections, can be detected with transvaginal sonography even several years following the Cesarean section [89] and their depth or size can be measured with saline infusion sonohysterography [90]. Further study is required to assess the risk of IUD use and pelvic inflammatory disease in Cesarean section ectopic pregnancy. Sonography is the first-line diagnostic tool for Cesarean scar pregnancy. Transvaginal ultrasound equipped with color Doppler imaging may serve as an additional tool to augment the diagnostic capabilities of transvaginal ultrasound; high-velocity, prominent, low-impedance blood flow can be detected surrounding an ectopic gestational sac, consistent with normal early pregnancy [91].

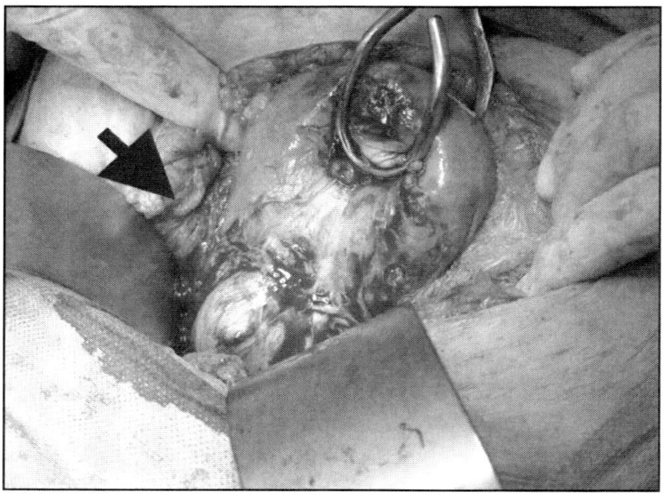

Figure 5. Cesarean scar Ectopic Pregnancy.

The early diagnosis of Cesarean scar pregnancy led to a high success rate of conservative treatment with local methotrexate administration alone [92, 93]. Direct local injection of methotrexate into the amniotic cavity of a Cesarean scar pregnancy using either transabdominal or transvaginal ultrasound-guided injection showed excellent outcomes [94. Local methotrexate administration increases the success rate due to the high concentration of methotrexate deposited in the lesion, avoiding the side effects produced with systemic administration [95].

Surgical or invasive techniques, including dilation and curettage, were not recommended for cesarean scar pregnancy due to high morbidity and poor prognosis, except for cases of failure of conservative treatment or rupture of the uterus due to delayed diagnosis.

Reports of pregnancy outcome after such an occurrence are rare. However, a subsequent pregnancy should be avoided for more than 3 months and probably 1 or 2 years.

For the pregnancy following a Cesarean scar pregnancy, it is preferable an early Cesarean section be done as soon as the fetal lungs become mature, to avoid the possibility of spontaneous uterine rupture.

Current Recruiting Clinical Trial on Management of Ectopic Pregnancy

- *Ectopic Trial: Laparascopy Versus Laparatomy in the Management of Ruptured Ectopic Pregnancy* University of Pretoria, *ClinicalTrials.gov Identifier: NCT01932957.*

  The trial will investigate the feasibility of treatment with laparoscopy and will look at outcomes such as hospital stay and pain experienced. The hypothesis is that laparoscopy is a feasible treatment option associated with shorter hospital stay and less pain.

- *KNC13-006: Methotrexate Treatment for Ectopic Pregnancy CHA University, ClinicalTrials.gov Identifier: NCT01855568*

  The purpose of this prospective randomized trial was to compare the success rates of single-dose and two-dose methotrexate protocol for the treatment of tubal ectopic pregnancy.

References

[1] Robson SJ, O'Shea RT. Undiagnosed ectopic pregnancy: a retrospective analysis of 31 "missed" ectopic pregnancies at a teaching hospital. *Aust. N. Z. J. Obstet. Gynaecol.,* 1996; 36:182-185.

[2] Stovall T et al. Emergency department diagnosis of ectopic pregnancy. *Ann. Emerg. Med.,* 1990; 19:1098-1103.

[3] Murray H et al. Diagnosis and treatment of ectopic pregnancy. *CMAJ,* 2005; 173: 905-912.

[4] Gracia CR, Barnhart KT. Diagnosing ectopic pregnancy: decision analysis comparing six strategies. *Obstet. Gynecol.,* 2001; 97: 464-70.

[5] Barnhart KT et al. Symptomatic patients with an early viable intrauterine pregnancy: HCG curves refined. *Obstet. Gynecol.,* 2004; 104: 50-5.

[6] Alkatout I. et al.; Clinical Diagnosis and Treatment of Ectopic Pregnancy. *Obstet. Gynecol. Survey,* 2013; 68: 571-581.

[7] Barnhart KT et al; Diagnostic accuracy of ultrasound above and below the beta-HCG discriminatory zone. *Obstet. Gynecol.,* 1999; 94: 583-587.

[8] Mol BW et al; Serum Human chorionic gonadotropin measurement in the diagnosis of ectopic pregnancy when transvaginal sonography is inconclusive. *Fertil. Steril.,* 1998; 70: 972-981.

[9] Kurjak A, Zalud I, Schulman H. Ectopic Pregnancy: transvaginal colo Doppler of trophoblastic flow in questionable adnexa. *J. Ultrasound. Med.,* 1991; 10: 685-689.

[10] Sivalingam VN, Duncan WC, Kirk E, et al. Diagnosis and management of ectopic pregnancy. *J. Fam. Plann. Reprod. Health Care,* 2011; 37: 231-240.

[11] Oron G., Tulandi T. A pragmatic and Evidence based Management of ectopic pregnancy. JMIG. 2013; 20: 446-454.

[12] Capmas P, Bouyer J, Fernandez H. Treatment of ectopic pregnancies in 2014: new answers to some old questions. *Fertil. Steril.,* 2014; 101: 615-620.

[13] Rabishong B. Predicting success of laparoscopic salpingostomy for ectopic pregnancy. *Obstet. Gynecol.,* 2010; 117:701-7.

[14] Kirk E, Van Calster B, Condous G et al. Ectopic pregnancy: using the HCG ratio to select women for expectant or medical management. *Acta Obstet. Gynecol. Scand.,* 2011; 90: 264-72.

[15] Van Mello NM, Mol F, Verhoeve HR et al. Methotrexate or expectant management in women with an ectopic pregnancy or pregnancy of

unknown location and low serum HCG concentrations? A randomized comparison. *Hum. Reprod.,* 2013; 28:60-7.

[16] Graczykowski JW, Mishell DR. Methotrexate prophylaxis for persistent ectopic pregnancy after conservative treatment by salpingostomy. *Obstet. Gynecol.,* 1997;89:118–22.

[17] Banerjee S, Aslam N, Woelfer B et al. Expectant management of early pregnancies of unknown location: a prospective evaluation of methods to predict spontaneous resolution od pregnancy. *BJOG,* 2001; 108: 158-63.

[18] Fernandez H, Yves Vincent SC, Pauthier S. Randomized trial of conservative laparoscopic treatment and methotrexate administrations in ectopic pregnancy and subsequent fertility. *Hum. Reprod.,* 1998; 13: 3239-43.

[19] Buster JE, Carson SA. Ectopic Pregnancy; new advances in diagnosis and treatment. *Curr. Opinion. Obstet. Gynecol.,* 1995; 7: 168-76.

[20] Akira S, Negishi Y, Abe T. et al., 2008. Prophylactic intratubal injection of methotrexate after linear salpingostomy for prevention of persistent ectopic pregnancy. *J. Obstet. Gynaecol. Res.,* 2008; 34: 885-9.

[21] Fernandez H. Capmas P. Lucot JP et al. Fertility after ectopic pregnancy: the DEMETER randomized tiral. Hum Reprod 2013; 28: 1247-53.

[22] Rajesh V, Lawrence M. Evidence based management of ectopic pregnancy. *Curr. Obstet. Gynecol.,* 2002;12:191-99.

[23] American College of Obstetrics and Gynecologists. ACOG Practice Bullettin n.94: medical management of ectopic pregnancy. *Obstet. Gynecol.,* 2008; 111: 1479.

[24] Da Costa Soares R, Elito J, Camano L. Increment in beta HVG in the 48 h period prior to treatment: a new variable predictive of therapeutic success in the treatment of ectopic pregnancy with methotrexate. *Arch. Gynecol. Obstet.,* 2008; 278: 319-24.

[25] Nowak-Markwitz E, Michalak M, Olejnik M et al. Cutoff value of human chorionic gonadotropin in relation to the number of methotrexate cycles in the successful treatment of ectopic pregnancy. *Fertil. Steril.,* 2009; 92: 1203-7.

[26] Tawfiq A, Agameya AF, Claman P. Predictors of treatment failure for ectopic pregnancy treated with single dose methotrexate. *Fertil. Steril.,* 2000; 74: 877-80.

[27] Moon MH, Lee YH, Lim KT et al. Outcome prediction for treatment of tubal pregnancy using an intramuscular methotrexate protocol. *J. Ultrasound. Med.,* 2008; 27: 1461-7.

[28] Menon S, Colins J, Barnhart KT. Establishing a human chorionic gonadotropin cutoff to guide methotrexate treatment of ectopic pregnancy: a systematic review. *Fertil. Steril.,* 2007; 87:481-4.

[29] Alleyassin A, Khademi A, Aghahosseini M et al. Comparison of success rates in the medical management of ectopic pregnancy with single dose and multiple dose administration of methotrexate: a prospective, randomized clinical trial. *Fertil. Steril.,* 2006; 85: 1661-1666.

[30] Guvendag Guven ES, Dilbaz S, Dilbaz B et al. Comparison of single and multiple dose methotrexate therapy for unruptured tubal ectopic pregnancy: a prospective randomized study. *Acta. Obstet. Gynecol. Scand.,* 2010; 89: 889-895.

[31] Hamed HO, Ahmed SR, Alghasham AA. Comparison of double and single dose methotrexate protocols for treatment of ectopis pregnancy. *Int. J. Gynecol. Obstet.,* 2012; 116:67-71.

[32] Weibel HS, Alserri A, Reinhold C. et al. Multidose methotrexate treatment of cervical pregnancy. *J. Obstet. Gynecol. Can.,* 2012; 34:359-62.

[33] Sivalingam VN, Duncan WC, Kirk E et al. Diagnosis and management of ectopic pregnancy. *J. Fam. Plann. Reprod. Health Care,* 2011; 37: 231-40.

[34] Kirk E, Condous G, Van Calster B. A validation of the most commonly used protocol to predict the success of single-dose methotrexate in the treatment of ectopic pregnancy. *Hum. Reprod.,* 2007; 22:858-63.

[35] K. Barnhart, A.C. Hummel, M.D. Sammel, S. Menon, J. Jain, N. Chakhtoura. Use of "2-dose" regimen of methotrexate to treat ectopic pregnancy. *Fertil. Steril.,* 87 (2007), pp. 250–256.

[36] Tawfiq, A.F. Agameya, P. Claman. Predictors of treatment failure for ectopic pregnancy treated with single-dose methotrexate. *Fertil. Steril.,* 74 (2000), pp. 877–880.

[37] M.B. Potter, L.A. Lepine, D.J. Jamieson. Predictors of success with methotrexate treatment of tubal ectopic pregnancy at Grady Memorial Hospital. *Am. J. Obstet. Gynecol.,* 188 (2003), pp. 1192–119.

[38] J. Elito Jr., A.P. Reichmann, M.N. Uchiyama, L. Camano. Predictive score for the systemic treatment of unruptured ectopic pregnancy with a single dose of methotrexate. *Int. J. Gynaecol. Obstet.,* 67 (1999), pp. 75–79.

[39] G.H. Lipscomb, K.J. Puckett, D. Bran, F.W. Ling. Management of separation pain after single-dose methotrexate therapy for ectopic pregnancy. *Obstet. Gynecol.,* 93 (1999), pp. 590–593.

[40] Alkatout I. Ectopic pregnancy. In: Schollmeyer T, et al. eds. Practical Manual for Laparoscopic & Hysteroscopic Gynecological Surgery. New Delhi, India: Jaypee Brothers Medical Publishers (P) Ltd; 2013: 169–189.
[41] Hucke J, Füllers U. Extrauterine Schwangerschaft. *Der Gynäkologe,* 2005; 6: 535–552.
[42] Lozeau AM, Potter B. Diagnosis and management of ectopic pregnancy. *Am. Fam. Physician.,* 2005; 72: 1707–1714.
[43] Lipscomb GH, Stovall TG, Ling FW. Nonsurgical treatment of ectopic pregnancy. *N. Engl. J. Med.,* 2000; 343: 1325–1329.
[44] Hoover KW, Tao G, Kent CK. Trends in the diagnosis and treatment of ectopic pregnancy in the United States. *Obstet. Gynecol.,* 115: 495–502
[45] Yao M, Tulandi T. Surgical and medical management of tubal and non-tubal ectopic pregnancies. *Curr. Opin. Obstet. Gynecol.,* 1998; 10: 371–374.
[46] Jermy K, Thomas J, Doo A, Bourne T. The conservative management of interstitial pregnancy. *BJOG,* 2004;111:1283–8.
[47] Fernandez H, Benifla JL, Madelenat P. Medical treatment of cornual pregnancy? *Fertil Steril,* 1996;66:862.
[48] Lau S, Tulandi T. Conservative medical and surgical management of interstitial ectopic pregnancy. *Fertil. Steril.,* 1999;72:207–15.
[49] 45. Kirk E, Bourne T. The nonsurgical management of ectopic pregnancy. *Curr. Opin. Obstet. Gynecol.,* 2006;18:587–93.
[50] Bourget P, Fernandez H, Quinquis-Desmaris V. Pharmacological treatment of ectopic pregnancy [article in French]. *Therapie,* 1993;48: 215–23.
[51] Timor-Tritsch IE. Hyperosmolar glucose injection for the treatment of heterotopic ovarian pregnancy. *Obstet. Gynecol.,* 2012;120:1212–3.
[52] Allison JL, Aubuchon M, Leasure JD, Schust DJ. Hyperosmolar glucose injection for the treatment of heterotopic ovarian pregnancy. *Obstet. Gynecol.,* 2012;120:449–52.
[53] Raughley MJ, Frishman GN. Local treatment of ectopic pregnancy. *Semin. Reprod. Med.,* 2007;25:99–115.
[54] Lang PF, Weiss PA, Mayer HO, Haas JG, Honigl W. Conservative treatment of ectopic pregnancy with local injection of hyperosmolar glucose solution or prostaglandin-F2 alpha: a prospective randomised study. *Lancet,* 1990; 336:78–81.

[55] Rock JA, Damario MA. Ectopic pregnancy. In: Rock JA, Jones HWIII, eds. Te-Linde's OperativeGynaecology. 9th ed. Philadelphia, PA: Lippincott Williams & Wilkins; 2003:507–536.

[56] Hung TH, Jeng CJ, Yang YC, et al. Treatment of cervical pregnancy with methotrexate. *Int. J. Gynecol. Obstet.,* 1996;53: 243–247.

[57] Ushakov FB, Elchalal U, Aceman PJ, et al. Cervical pregnancy: past and future. *Obstet. Gynecol. Surv.,* 1997;52:45–59.

[58] Wolcott HD, Kaunitz AM, Nuss RC, et al. Successful pregnancy after previous conservative treatment of an advanced cervical pregnancy. *Obstet. Gynecol.,* 1998;71:1023–1025.

[59] Shinagawa S, Nagayama M. Cervical pregnancy as a possible sequel of induced abortion. *Am. J. Obstet. Gynecol.,* 1969;105: 282–284.

[60] Rothe DJ, Birnbaum SJ. Cervical pregnancy. *Obstet. Gynecol.,* 1973;42: 675–680.

[61] Dicker D, Feldberg D, Samuel N, et al. Etiology of cervical pregnancy. *J. Reprod. Med.,* 1985;30:25–27.

[62] Paalman RJ, McElin TW. Cervical pregnancy. Review of the literature and presentation of cases. *Am. J. Obstet. Gynecol.,* 1959;77:1261.

[63] Raskin MM. Diagnosis of cervical pregnancy by ultrasound: a case report. *Am. J. Obstet. Gynecol.,* 1978;130:234–235.

[64] Jurkovic D, Hacket E, Campbell S. Diagnosis and treatment of early cervical pregnancy. A reviewand a report of two cases treated conservatively. *Ultrasound Obstet. Gynecol.,* 1996;8:373–380.

[65] Bader-Armstrong B, Shah Y, Rubens D. Use of ultrasound and magnetic resonance imaging in the diagnosis of cervical pregnancy. *J. Clin. Ultrasound.,* 1989;17:283–286.

[66] Farabow W, Fulton J, Fletcher V Jr, et al. Cervical pregnancy treated with methotrexate. *N. C. Med. J.,* 1983;44:91–93.

[67] Song MJ, Moon MH, Kim JA, et al. Serial transvaginal sonographic findings of cervical ectopic pregnancy treated with high-dose methotrexate. *J. Ultrasound. Med.,* 2009;28:55–61.

[68] Dall P, Pfisterer J, Du Bois A, et al. Therapeutic strategies in cervical pregnancy. *Eur. J. Obstet. Gynecol. Reprod. Biol.,* 1994; 56:195–200.

[69] Spitzer D, Steiner H, Graf A, et al. Conservative treatment of cervical pregnancy by curettage and local prostaglandin injection. *Hum. Reprod.,* 1997;12;860–866.

[70] Kim JS, Nam KH, Kim TH, et al. Hysteroscopic management of cervical pregnancy with intrauterine irrigation with H2O2. *J. Minim. Invasive Gynecol.,* 2008;15:627–630.

[71] Shrestha E, Yang Y, Li X, et al. Successful conservative management with methotrexate and mifepristone of cervical pregnancy. *J. Biomed. Res.,* 2011;25:71–73.

[72] Jurkovic D, Hacket E, Campbell S. Diagnosis and treatment of early cervical pregnancy. A reviewand a report of two cases treated conservatively. *Ultrasound Obstet. Gynecol.,* 1996;8:373–380.

[73] Lobel SM, Meyerovitz MF, Benson CC, et al. Preoperative angiographic uterine artery embolization in the management of cervical pregnancy. *Obstet. Gynecol.,* 1990;76:938–941.

[74] Kung FT, Lin H, Hsu TY, et al. Differential diagnosis of suspected cervical pregnancy and conservative treatment with the combination of laparoscopy-assisted uterine artery ligation and hysteroscopic endocervical resection. *Fertil Steril.,* 2004;81;1642–1649.

[75] Tulandi T, AL-Jaroudi D. Interstitial pregnancy: results generated from the society of Reproductive Surgeons Registry. *Obstet. Gynecol.,* 2004;103:47–50.

[76] Rock JA, Thompson JD (eds). Telinde's operative gynecology, 8th edn. Philadelphia, PA: *Lippincott-Raven,* 1997:505–20.

[77] Stovall TG, Ling FW. Single dose methotrexate: a clinical trial. *Am. J. Obstet. Gynecol.,* 1993;168:1759–65.

[78] Weissman A, Fishman A. Uterine rupture following conservative surgery for interstitial pregnancy. *Eur. J. Obstet. Gynecol. Reprod. Biol.,* 1992;60:428–32.

[79] Benifla JL, Fernandez H, Sebban E, Darai E, Frydman R, Medelanet P. Alternative to surgery of treatment of unruptured interstitial pregnancy: 15 cases of medical treatment. *Eur. J. Obstet. Gynecol. Reprod. Biol.,* 1996;70:151– 6.

[80] Moon HS, Choi YJ, Park YH, Kim SG. New simple endoscopic operation for interstitial pregnancies. *Am. J. Obstet. Gynecol.,* 2000;182: 114–21.

[81] Lau S, Tulandi T. Conservative medical and surgical management of interstitial ectopic pregnancy. *Fertil. Steril.,* 1999;72:207–15.

[82] Meyer W, Mitchell D. Hysteroscopic removal of an interstitial ectopic gestation. A case report. *J. Reprod. Med.,* 1989;34:928–9.

[83] Soriano D, Vicus D, Mashiach R, Sciff E, Seidman D, Goldenberg M. Laparoscopic treatment of corneal pregnancy: a series of 20 consecutive cases. *Fertil Steril,* 2007;11:1–5.

[84] Chan LY, Fok WY, Yuen PM. Pitfall in the diagnosis of interstitial pregnancy. *Acta. Obstet. Gynecol. Scand.,* 2003;82:867–70.

[85] Jermy K, Thomas J, Doo A, Bourne T. The conservative treatment of interstitial pregnancy. *Br. J. Obstet. Gynaecol.,* 2004;111:1283–8.

[86] Reich H, Johns DA, DeCaprio J, McGlynn F, Reich E. Laparoscopic treatment of 109 consecutive ectopic pregnancies. *J. Reprod. Med.,* 1988;33:885–90

[87] Picardo E et al., Acute abdomen in interstitial ectopic pregnancy, an emergency laparoscopic treatment. Case Reports in Womens Health doi: 10.1016/j.crwh.2014.06.002 in press.

[88] Godin PA, Bassil S, Donnez J. An ectopic pregnancy developing in a previous cesarean section scar. *Fertil. Steril.,* 1997; 67:398–400.

[89] Chen HY, Chen SJ, Hsieh FJ. Observation of cesarean section scar by transvaginal ultrasonography. *Ultrasound Med. Biol.,* 1990; 16: 443–447.

[90] Monteagudo A, Carreno C, Timor-Tritsch IE. Saline infusion sonohysterography in nonpregnant women with previous cesarean delivery: the "niche" in the scar. *J. Ultrasound. Med.,* 2001; 20: 1105–1115.

[91] Jurkovic D, Jauniaux E, Kurjak A, Hustin J, Campbell S, Nicolaides KH. Transvaginal color Doppler assessment of the uteroplacental circulation in early pregnancy. *Obstet. Gynecol.,* 1991; 77: 365–369.

[92] Feichtinger W, Kemeter P. Conservative treatment of ectopic pregnancy by transvaginal aspiration under sonographic control and methotrexate injection. *Lancet,* 1987; 1: 381–382.

[93] Yankowitz J, Leake J, Huggins G, Gazaway P, Gates E. Cervical ectopic pregnancy: Review of the literature and report of a case treated by single dose methotrexate therapy. *Obstet. Gynecol. Surv.,* 1990; 45: 405–414.

[94] Seow KM, Cheng WC, Chuang J, Lee C, Tsai YL, Hwang JL. Methotrexate for cesarean scar pregnancy following in vitro fertilization and embryo transfer: A case report. *J. Reprod. Med.,* 2000; 45: 754–757.

[95] Schiff E, Shalev E, Bustan M, Tsabari M,Mashiach S,Weiner E. Pharmacokinetics of methotrexate after local tubal injection for conservative treatment of ectopic pregnancy. *Fertil. Steril.,* 1992; 57: 688–690.

In: Ectopic Pregnancy
Editor: Mallory T. Church
ISBN: 978-1-63463-260-7

Chapter 4

Cervical Ectopic Pregnancy

José C. Maañón Di Leo [*]
Department of Obstetrics & Gynaecology, Marbella, Málaga, Spain

Abstract

Cervical ectopic pregnancy is a rare complication of gestation, and it accounts for less than 1 % of all ectopic pregnancies, with a reported incidence of 1 in 1000-95.000 pregnancies.

From the moment that ultrasound plays a crucial role in the diagnosis of cervical ectopic pregnancy and its differential diagnosis with abortion, the chapter pays special attention to the ultrasound diagnosis criteria.

Medical treatment of cervical ectopic pregnancy with methotrexate is well established and is widely accepted as the primary treatment. Treatment with methotrexate is effective in many cases, but in some cases pregnancy reaches 9 or more weeks. In these cases it is necessary to use other therapeutic tools to increase success rates.

The chapter also reviews the predictors of treatment failure.

Finally the chapter provides an algorithm on how to associate the different treatment options.

Keywords: Cervical ectopic pregnancy

---

[*] Corresponding author: Urb. Las Dunas Beach Block 2A portal 11, Las Chapas, Marbella, Málaga, Spain, Telephone number: 0034- 952835050, E – mail: jcm_4400@yahoo.com.

Introduction

Cervical ectopic pregnancy (CEP) is a rare complication of gestation, and it accounts for less than 1 % of all ectopic pregnancies, with a reported incidence of 1 in 1000-95.000 pregnancies. Although maternal morbidity is still high, the mortality rate has declined during the 20th century to near zero today (Faschingbauer 2011).

Even the widespread use of ultrasound, its diagnosis was rarely made before curettage (Kirk 2006). The first report of a cervical ectopic pregnancy diagnosed using ultrasound was in 1978 (Raskin 1978).

The reproductive function is usually preserved by means of a satisfactory conservative treatment (Celik 2003). Unfortunately, hysterectomy is sometimes necessary due to an untreatable haemorrhage (Hung 1996).

Risk Factors

The aetiology of cervical ectopic pregnancy is unclear, suspected mechanism is damage of the cervix during operative uterine procedures like caesarean section (Capini 2004, Kochi 2014, Chrestiana 2014), prior uterine curettage, induced abortion, Ascherman´s sindrome, use of intrauterine device. Other risk factors are prior exposure in uterus to diethylsstilbesterol, congenital structural uterine abnormalities, large uterine fibroids, infection or inflammation, advanced maternal age and the development and increasing use of assisted reproductive technologies.

Indeed, have been described cases of cervical twin ectopic pregnancies after in vitro embryo transfer (Aboulfoutouh 2011).

This factors may be interfere with the blastocys implantation and retard the pass and implantation of blastocys at the cervix (Shan 2014).

Diagnosis

In the last decades, the greater accessibility to the transvaginal ultrasound, and the widespread use of the beta human chorionic gonadotropin (b hCG), has allowed that most of the ectopic pregnancies, including the cases of cervical ectopic pregnancies are diagnosed early.

As a result of earlier diagnosis patients have minors serum b hCG levels, are clinically more stable and have more possibilities of carrying out a conservative treatment.

The most common clinical sing is vaginal bleeding, and de speculum examination will reveal vaginal bleeding but be otherwise unremarkable.

Bimanual examinations reveal a disproportionately soft and large cervix (like a barrel shape) in relation with de gestational age. Sometimes is possible see fetal tissue thought the cervical os, which appears purple. Exploration may cause sever haemorrhage.

First trimester vaginal bleeding associated o not with pelvic pain is a common reason for emergency department consultation (Chrestiana 2014, Shavell 2012). CEP can be taken wrongly as an intra uterine pregnancy or an abortion.

The reported accuracy of transvaginal ultrasound in diagnosis CEP is near to 88% (Kochi 2014)

Currently the diagnosis of CEP is performed following these ultrasounds criteria (Timor 1994, Ushakov 1997, Sarita 2006, Pereira 2013): 1) an empty hourglass shaped uterus 2) a barrel shape cervix 3) gestational sac present below de level of the uterine arteries 4) an intact portion of the cervical canal between the gestational sac and the endometrium 5) absence of the sliding sing (applied pressure to the cervix with de vaginal probe, in case de spontaneous abortion the gestational sac slides against de endocervical canal) and 6) using colour Doppler is possible identify sings suggestive of cervical implantation or local invasion of the endocervical tissue by the trophobalst: high velocity and low impedance blow flow. Figure 1, 2, 3.

The diagnosis is much easier to make when there is visible fetal cardiac activity, which usually excludes cervical abortion, nevertheless with the use of home urinary pregnancy tests for diagnosis and with the availability of transvaginal ultrasound, cervical pregnancies may therefore be diagnosed early, when only the gestational sac without yolk sac or fetal pole is visible

Ander these principia, most CEP are diagnosed between 37 – 70 days of gestation (Wang 2011).

Magnetic resonance (MRI) was also used in the diagnosis of CEP, and could be helpful when de diagnosis is not clear. MRI findings are and ill – marinated mass with an heterogeneous signal intensity on T2 – weighted images, irregular internal high signal intensities on T1 - weighted images, and a circumferential rim of low signal intensity (Kochi 2014).

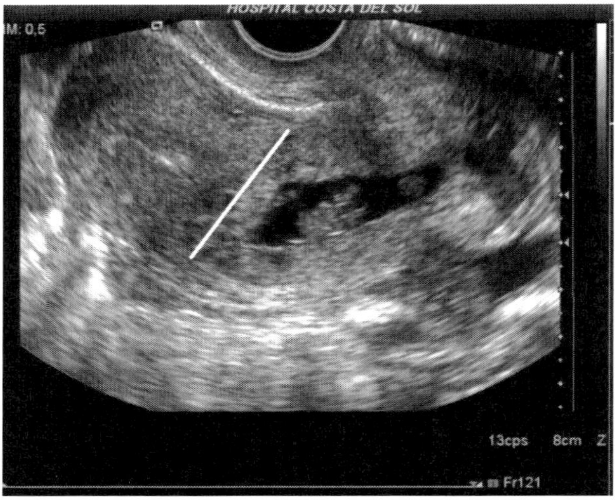

Figure 1. Ultrasound diagnosis criteria. Gestational sac present below de level of the uterine arteries. Comment bottom picture: line al the level of internal os.

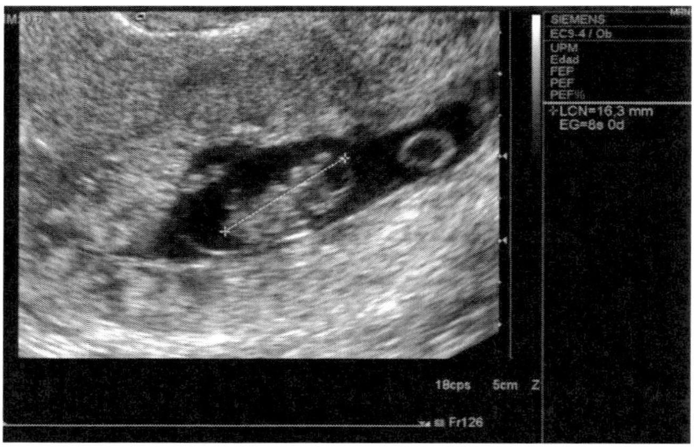

Figure 2. Ultrasound diagnosis criteria. An intact portion of the cervical canal between the gestational sac and the endometrium.

Sonographic appearance is of great importance to avoid confusion with other diseases (Ahmadi 2012) (Table I).

In case of spontaneous abortion the gestational sac appears deformed without the characteristic echogenic ring. By gentle pressure of the probe is possible to show that the products of conception are moved, which is called the sliding sing. Color doppler does not demonstrate a “ring of fire”.

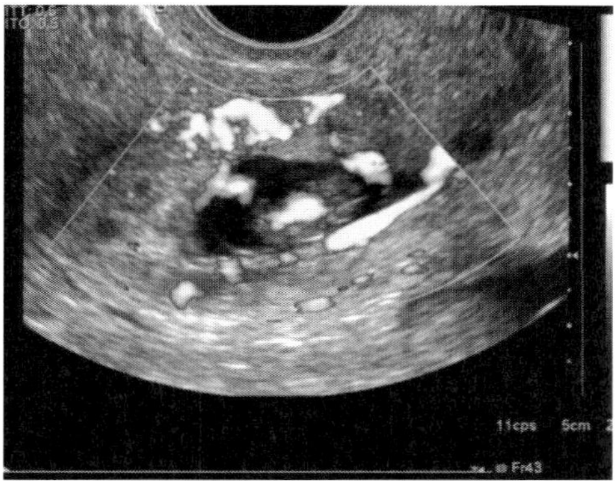

Figure 3. Ultrasound diagnosis criteria. Ring of fire.

There have also been described sonographic signs that distinguish between CEP and pregnancy in the caesarean scar. The history of a previous cesarean section and thinning of the myometrium can be seen near the bladder.

Nabothian cys (Modayil 2011) are well circumscribed anechoic structures, are not isolated, and has posterior echogenic enhancement. Color doppler show a high resistance peripheral flow.

The value of beta hCG discriminatory level in the diagnosis and management of CEP is not clear, and can not be used in the same way that for pregnancies of unknown location (Ngu 2013).

Olso, there are rare cases of intramural CEP (Ohtsuka 2012, Taskim 2009, Kirk 2009)

There are also pathologic diagnostic criteria (Cipullo 2008): 1) cervical glands opposite the placental attachment 2) trophobalst intimately attach to the cervix and situated below the level of uterine vessels 3) uterine cavity without fetal tissue (Parente 1983).

Treatment

Methotrexate

Management options for cervical pregnancies range from conservative treatments (drug therapies) to radical surgical procedures (El – Matary 2005) and there is no single strategy recognized as the standard for the treatment of CEP.

Table I. Ultrasound criteria for diagnosis of CEP a differential diagnosis from other pathologies

Diagnosis	Criteria
Interstitial CEP	· Empty uterine cavity · Conception products outside endometrial layer and surrounded by miometrium
CEP	· An empty hourglass shaped uterus · A barrel shape cervix · Gestational sac present below de level of the uterine arteries · An intact portion of the cervical canal between the gestational san and the endometrium · Absence of the sliding sing (apllied pressure to the cervix with de vaginal probe, in case de spontaneous abortion the gestational sac slides against de endocervical canal) and · Color Doppler is possible identify sings suggestive of cervical implantation or local invasion od the endocervical tissue by the trophobalst: high velocity and low impedance bloow flow.
EP in caesarean section scar	· Empty uterus · Gestational sac al the lever of caesarean scar · Sliding sing absent · Positive Doppler circulation
Abortion	· The gestational sac appears deformed without the characteristic echogenic ring. · By gentle pressure of the probe is possible to show that the products of conception are moved, which is called the sliding sing. · Color doppler does not demonstrate a "ring of fire
Naboth cyst	· Well circumscribed anechoic structures, not isolated · Posterior echogenic enhancement. · Color doppler show a high resistance peripheral flow.

The general principles in the management of CEP are minimize blood loss, remove products of conception, and fertility preservation (Bianchi 2011).

The fact that most of the patients came from assisted reproductive treatments, in a sub fertile population, makes more likely that theses patients desires fertility preservation (Moragiani 2012).

Probably the most challenging cases are heterotopic pregnancies, which pose the problem of preserving orthotopic gestation (Bianchi 2011).

Before 12 weeks of gestation, the invasion of trophoblastic tissue of the cervix wall is not sufficiently deep, then the possibility to obtain successful results using conservative treatment is greater.

Treatment with MTX, a flolic acid antagonist, was established in the late 1980 and achieved results comparable with surgery when it is used in the treatment of common ectopic pregnancies (Ory 1983).

Historically the best candidates for medical management of ectopic pregnancies with MTX patients with hemodynamic stability, with not severe pelvic pain and normal baseline liver and renal function tests (ASRM 2008).

Then just before the first dose of MTX, patients should be screened with blood count, liver and renal function test, blood type and Rh.

Two treatment regimens have been the most used.

Multiple dose protocol was adapted form the treatment for trophoblastic disease. This protocol alternates MTX (1mg/kg) with leucovorin (0,1 mg / kg) (Gutierrez 2012). The protocol is carry on until hCG falls by 15% from de mayor concentration. Olmost 50% of the patient not need to complete the protocol (Table II).

A second regime is named single dose and was described by Stovall. In this protocol MTX is administrated by a single injection of MTX 50 mg / m2 via IM.

There have been no direct comparison between this two alternatives, but one meta analysis including 26 articles showed an overall treatment success of 89%, even if the multiple dose regimen have a success rate of 92.7% witch was statistically higher than that achieved with the monodose.

We must remember that these protocols were designed fist for the treatment of trophoblastic disease and then applied to tubal ectopic pregnancy, none of them was specifically designed to treat CEP.

Same thing happens with predictive factors related to MTX treatment success. Theses factors were described for de treatment of tubal ectopic pregnancy.

Predictive factors for success in case of CEP should be different.

Conservative treatment of CEP usually works only in cases diagnosed before 12 week (Alkatout 2013). Hung el al., after compiled 52 cases from 28 publications inferred that the chance of failure increase if the following factors are present: 1) gestational age > 9 weeks 2) beta hCG level > 10,000 mIU/mL, positive fetal cardiac activity and crown rump length > 10 mm (Chaudhary 2013, Adabi 2013 Chetty 2009).

MTX has been used with de addition of mifepristone 600 mg (Gómez 2012). The combination of the two drugs produced a rapid cell lysis. The more impressing results were obtained when level of serum progesterone were >10ng/ml.

Table II. Multiple dose protocol

Treatment day	test	intervention
1	hCG + blood test + liver and renal function + blood type	MTX 1.0 mg / kg IM
2		Leu 0,1 mg / kg IM
3	hCG	MTX 1.0 mg / kg IM. If < 15% decline day 1 to day 3 If > 15% decine, stop treatment and start Fw - Up
4		Leu 0,1 mg / kg IM
5	hCG	MTX 1.0 mg / kg IM. If < 15% decline day 3 to day 5 If > 15% decine, stop treatment and start Fw - Up
6		Leu 0,1 mg / kg IM
7	hCG	MTX 1.0 mg / kg IM. If < 15% decline day 5 to day 7 If > 15% decine, stop treatment and start Fw - Up
8		Leu 0,1 mg / kg IM

MTX = metotrexate, Leuc = leucovorin, IM = intra muscular.

MTX also used by injection into uterine arteries with de aim of fertility preservation (Kochi 2014) performed a percutaneous access of the femoral arteries with a flexible angiographic catheter and injected 50 mg to each uterine artery. Is important to note that one patient necessitated subsequent artery embolization.

Finally, MTX has also been used by ultrasound guided intra amniotic injection with o without potassium chloride (Sijanovic 2011). Intra amniotic MTX has been proven more efficient in 9 weeks of gestational age.

Following single dose protocol, some authors proposed different scenarios according to the levels of b hCG measured on day 4. For example if b hCG levels showed slight changes and ultrasound shows no gestational sac, an expectant attitude is taken to obtain the values on day 7. If however, persistence of gestational sac is observed with increase of peripheral vascularisation or hCG levels were significantly increased, uterine artery embolization and vacuum is performed (Gomez 2012).

Potassium Chloride Use

Potassium chloride (KCl) use in CEP was reported in a number of case series and is a reasonable approach to initial treatment MTX / Leu with o without uterine artery embolization (UAE) (Morgan 2013, Zakaria 2011). KCl is use by intra amniotic injection with the idea to produce cardioplegia and further cell division and improve therapeutics results. This option is safe and useful in cases of heterotrophic pregnancies.

Unfortunately the use of KCl associated with UAE in a small number of cases does not reveal whether it is a necessary component in the resolution CEP.

Curettage and Ballon Tamponade

Curettage and ballon tamponade has been used after administration of methotrexate with successful results (Bakour 2005).

This option permit treats heterotopic CEP with ultrasound guided curettage, leaving the intrauterine pregnancy intact.

Another possibility of using this procedure is in case of acute haemorrhage related to residual CEP (Pereira 2013).

Recently Flystra (Flystra 2014) in a series of 13 cases of CEP demonstrated that suction curettage was 100% successful in terminating fist trimester CEP.

The technique starts with a circumferential infiltration of cervical stoma around de CEP with 20 ml of diluted vasopressin. This step was followed by the placement of an untied Mc Donald cerclaje, read to tie in case of hemorrhagic problems.

Curetagge was performed with an suction curettage with a diameter equal of the gestational age in weeks and without cervical canal dilation. Immediately after a balloon was placed into de cervical canal and inflated, and left in place for 24 hour. Sharp curettage was avoided.

Uterine Artery Embolization

This treatment option is usually applicable in conditions of acute massive hemorrhage, positive fetal cardiac activity, high initial levels of hCG (> 10 000 IU / mL or 34,000 IU/mL (ZaKaria 2011)) and higher gestational ages of 8-9 weeks (Wang 2011), factors that resulted in a high failure rate of the medical treatment with MTX or require an immediate action. Another advantage is a one step procedure.

Using digital angiography and going through the right femoral artery, a catheter is inserted to reach the uterine arteries. Usually, after making the bilateral embolization, the procedure ends by performing a vacuum evacuation under ultrasound control. Wang et al. reported a series of cases, with an average time of 40 minutes per procedure and blood loss averaged 27ml without serious complications occurred. Complete regression occurred at a median time of 39 days.

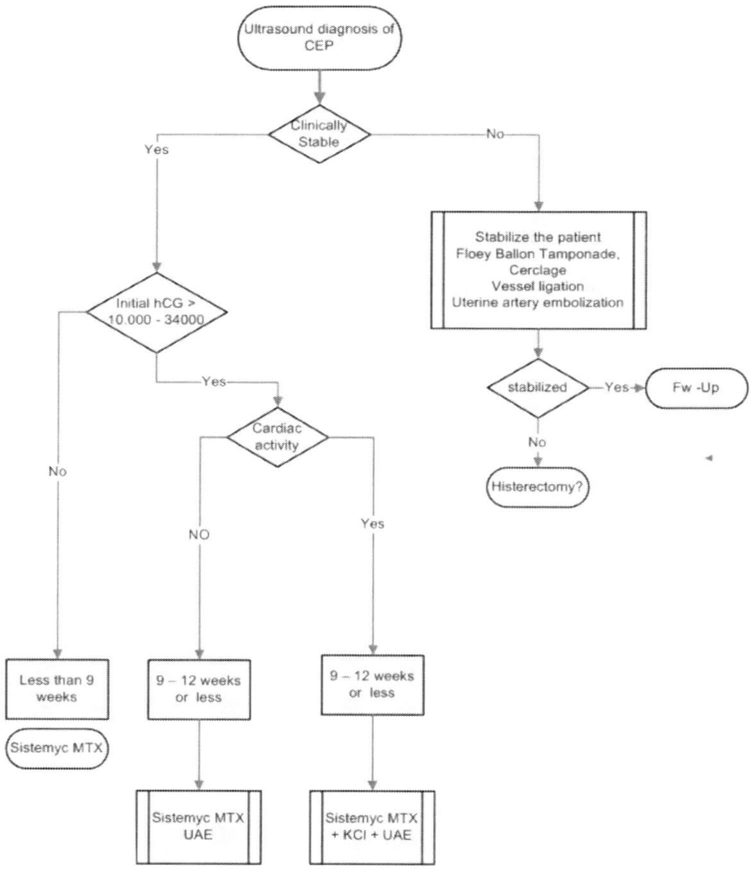

Figure 4. treatment flow chart. MTX: methotrexate, UAE: uterine artery embolization, KCL: potassium chloride.

The uses of an evacuation vacuum is used to prevent a quickly restored of collateral circulation in the cervix.

UAE can be repeated in case of a new vaginal bleeding occurs. The residual trophoblastic tissue may regrow after a new establishing collateral circulation. The presence of positive fetal cardiac activity prior to the start of the first treatment is a risk factor for late vaginal bleeding, this cases can be treated by UAE (Hirakawa 2009).

In cases of severe acute uterine haemorrhage bilateral uterine artery embolization has been recently used in association with systemic methotrexate (Sherer 2003).

Conclusion

Units of Obstetrics & Gynecology should be able to offer different types of conservative treatments for ectopic cervical pregnancy. Conservative medical treatment of cervical ectopic pregnancy whit methotrexate is safe and effective. The essential is to reach a fast and accurate diagnosis by means of bHcg levels and trasvaginal ultrasound.

References

Aboulfoutouh, II; Youssef, MAF; Zakaria, AE; Mady, AAF; Khattab, SM. Cervical twin ectopic pregnancy after In Vitro fertilization-Embryo transfer (IVF-ET): case report. *Gynecological Endocrinology*, December 2011, 27(12): 1007–1009.

Adabi, K; Nekuie, S; Rezaeei, Z; Rahimi-Sharbaf, F; Banifatemi, S; Salimi, S. Conservative management of cervical ectopic pregnancy: systemic methotrexate followed by curettage. *Arch Gynecol Obstet*, (2013) 288, 687–689.

Ahmadi, F; Irani, S. Cervical Ectopic Pregnancy following Assisted Reproductive Technology: A Case Report. *Royan Institute International Journal of Fertility and Sterility*, Vol 6, No 3, Oct-Dec, 2012, 201-204.

Alkatout, I; Honemeyer, U; Alexander, Strauss, A; Tinelli, A; Malvasi, A; Walte, J; Mettler, L. Schollmeyer Clinical Diagnosis and Treatment of Ectopic Pregnancy. *Obstetrical and gynecological survey.*, Volume 68, Number 8, 571 – 581.

American Society for Reproductive Medicine, Birmingham, Alabama. Medical treatment of ectopic pregnancy: a committee opinión. *Fertil Steril*, 2008, 90, S206–12.

Bakour, SH; Thompson, PK; Khan, KS. Successful conservative management of cervical ectopic pregnancy with combination of methotrextate, mifepristone, surgical evacuation and tamponade using a double balloon three-way catheter. *J Obstet Gynaecol.*, 2005, 25(6), 616-8.

Bianchi, P; Salvatori, MM; Torcia, F; Cozza, G; Mossa, B. Cervical pregnancy. *Fertil Steril*, 2011, 95, 2123.e3–e4.

Capini, I; Ocal, P; Erkan, S; Erzik, B. Conservative treatment of cervical ectopic pregnancy with transvaginal ultrasound guided aspiration and single dose methotrexate. *Fertil Steril*, 2004, 81(4), 1130-1132.

Celik, C; Bala, A; Acar, A; Gezginc, K; Akyurek, C. Methotrexate for cervical pregnancy. A case report. J Reprod Med., 2003, 48(2), 130-2.

Chaudhary, V; Sachdeva, P; Kumar, D; Arora, R; Banavaliker, J. Khan M. Conservative management of cervical pregnancy A repost of two cases. *J Reprod Med*, 2013, 58, 451 – 457.

Chrestiana, D; Cheng, AB; Panebianco, NL,Anthony, J. Dean AJ.Pitfalls in cervical ectopic pregnancy diagnosis by emergency physicians using bedside ultrasonography. *American Journal of Emergency Medicine*, 32 (2014) 397.e1–397.e3.

Chetty, M; Elson, J. Treating non-tubal ectopic pregnancy. *Best Practice & Research Clinical Obstetrics and Gynaecology*, 23, (2009) 529–538.

Cipullo, L; Cassese, S; Fasolino, L; Fasolino, MC,Fasolino, A. Cervical pregnancy: A case series and a review of current clinical practice. *The European Journal of Contraception and Reproductive Health Care*, September, 2008, 13(3), 313–319.

El-Matary, AM; Ashworth, F. Cervical ectopic pregnancy with successful conservative treatment. *J Obstet Gynaecol.*, 2005, 25(4), 411-2.

Faschingbauer, F; Muelle, A; Voigt, F; Beckman, MW; Goecke, TW. Treatment of heterotopic cervical pregnancies. *Fertil Steril*, 2011, 95, 1787.e9–e13.

Fylstra, DL. Cervical pregnancy: 13 cases treated with suction curettage and balloon tamponade. *Am J Obstet Gynecol*, 2014, 210, 581.e1-5.

Gómez, García MT; Aguarón, Benitez G; Barberá, Belda B; Callejón, Rodríguez C; González, Merlo G. Medical therapy (methotrexate and mifepristone) alone or in combination with another type of therapy for the management of cervical or interstitial ectopic pregnancy. *European*

Journal of Obstetrics & Gynecology and Reproductive Biology, 2012, 165, 77–81.

Gosakan, R; Arutchelvam, S; Gergis, HH; Emovon, E. Medical management of a cervical ectopic pregnancy. *J Obstet Gynaecol.*, 2005, 25(1), 82-3.

Hirakawa, M; Tajima, T; Yoshimitsu, K; Irie, H; Ishigami, K; Yahata, H; Wake, N; Honda, H. Uterine Artery Embolization Along With the Administration of Methotrexate for Cervical Ectopic Pregnancy: Technical and Clinical Outcomes. *AJR*, 2009, 192, 1601–1607.

Hung, TH; Jeng, CJ; Yang, YC; Wang, KG; Lan, CC. Treatment of cervical pregnancy with methotrexate. *Int J Gynaecol Obstet.*, 1996, 53(3), 243-7.

Kirk, E; Condous, G; Haider, Z; Syed, A; Ojha, K; Bourne, T. The conservative management of cervical ectopic pregnancies. *Ultrasound Obstet Gynecol.*, 2006, 27(4), 430-7.

Kirk, E; Bourne, T. Diagnosis of ectopic pregnancy with ultrasound. *Best Practice & Research Clinical Obstetrics and Gynaecology*, 2009, 23, 501–508.

Kochi, K; Hidaka, T; Yasoshima, K; Yoneda, K; Arai, K, and, Arai, T. Cervical pregnancy: A report of four cases. *J. Obstet. Gynaecol.*, Res. Vol. 40, No. 2, 603–606.

Marín, Gutiérrez A; Garrido, Luque B; García, Martín L; Benítez, Toledo L; Maañón, di Leo JC. Tratamiento del embarazo ectópico cervical con metotrexato y rescate con leucovorina. *Prog Obstet Ginecol.*, 2011, 54(7), 379—382.

Modayil, V; Ash, A; Raio, C. Cervical ectopic pregnancy diagnosed by point-of-care emergency Department ultrasound. *The Journal of Emergency Medicine*, 2011, Vol. 41, No. 6, 655–657.

Moragianni, VA; Hamar, BD; Colin, McArdle, C, David, A. Ryley CDA. Management of a cervical heterotopic pregnancy presenting with first-trimester bleeding: case report and review of the literatura. *Fertil Steril*, 2012, 98, 89–94.

Ngu, SF; Ko, JKY; Cheung, VYT. Value of human chorionic gonadotropin levels in diagnosing cervical ectopic pregnancy. *Acta Obstetricia et Gynecologica Scandinavica*, 2013, 92, 608–609.

Ohtsuka, T; Hirata, T; Tsukiyama, T; Takana, H; Kawaguchi, H; Terao, K. A very rare case of an ectopic cervical intramural Pregnancy. *Fertil Steril*, 2011, 95, 291.e11–e13.

Ory, SJ; Villanueva, AL; Sand, PK; et al. Conservative treatment of actopic pregnancy with methotrexate. *Am J Obstet Gynecol*, 1986, 154(6), 1299-306.

Parente, JT; OU, CS; Levy, el al. Cervical pregnancy analysis: A review and report of five cases. *Obstet Gynecol*, 1983, 62 (1), 79-82.

Raskin, MM. Diagnosis of cervical pregnancy by ultrasound. A case report. *Am J Obstet Gynecol*, 1978, 130, 234-235.

Shavell, VI; Abdallah, ME; Zakaria, MA; Berman, JM; Diamond, MP; Elizabeth, E., Puscheck, EE. Misdiagnosis of cervical ectopic pregnancy. *Arch Gynecol Obstet*, (2012) 285, 423–426.

Sherer, DM; Lysikiewicz, A; Abulafia, O. Viable cervical pregnancy managed with systemic methotrexate, uterine artery embolization, and local tamponade with inflated Foley catheter balloon. *Am J Perinatol.*, 2003, 20(5), 263-7.

Swank, ML; Harken, TR; Porto, M.Management of Interstitial Ectopic Pregnancies With a Combined Intra-Amniotic and Systemic Approach. *Obstet Gynecol*, 2013, 122, 461–4).

Pereira, N; Grias, I; Foster, SE; Della, Badia, CR. Acute Hemorrhage Related to a Residual Cervical Pregnancy: Management with Curettage, Tamponade, and Cerclage. *Journal of Minimally Invasive Gynecology*, (2013) 20, 907–911.

Starita, A; Di Miscia, A; Evangelista, S; Donadio, F; Starita, A. Cervical ectopic pregnancy: clinical review. *Clin Exp Obstet Gynecol.*, 2006, 33(1), 47-9.

Shan, N; Don, D; Deng, W, and, Fu, Y. Unusual ectopic pregnancies: A retrospective analysis of 65 cases. *J. Obstet. Gynaecol. Res.*, Vol. 40, No. 1, 147–154.

Sijanovic, S; Vidosavljevic, D; Ivanka, Sijanovic I. Methotrexate in local treatment of cervical heterotopic pregnancy with successful perinatal outcome: Case report. *J. Obstet. Gynaecol. Res.*, Vol. 37, No. 9, 1241–1245.

Taskın, S; Elif, Aylin; Taskın, EA; Cengiz, B. Cervical intramural ectopic pregnancy. *Fertil Steril*, 2009, 92, 395.e5–e7.

Timor-Tritsch, IE; Monteagudo, A; Mandeville, EO; Peisner, DB; Anaya, GP; Pirrone, EC. Successful management of viable cervical pregnancy by local injection of methotrexate guided by transvaginal ultrasonography. *Am J Obstet Gynecol*, 1994, 170, 737-9.

Ushakov, FB; Elchalal, U; Aceman, PJ; Schenker, JG. Cervical pregnancy: past and future. *Obstetrical and Gynecological Survey*, 1997, 52, 45–59.

Wang, Y; Xu, B; Dai, S; et al. An efficient conservative treatment modality for cervical pregnancy: angiographic uterine artery embolization followed by immediate curettage. *Am J Obstet Gynecol*, 2011, 204, 31.e1-7.

Zakaria, MA; Abdallah, ME; Shavell, VI; Jay, M. Berman JM, Diamond MP, Kmak DC.Conservative management of cervical ectopic pregnancy: utility of uterine artery embolization. *Fertil Steril*, 2011, 95, 872–6.

In: Ectopic Pregnancy
Editor: Mallory T. Church
ISBN: 978-1-63463-260-7

Chapter 5

Ectopic Pregnancy: Diagnosis and Treatment

***Fa-Tsai Wang*[1] *and Chi-Wen Juan*[1,2,*]**
[1]Department of Emergency Medicine,
Kuang Tien General Hospital, Taichung, Taiwan (R.O.C.)
[2]Department of Nursing, Hungkuang University, Taichung, Taiwan (R.O.C.)

Abstract

Ectopic pregnancy occurs when the developing blastocyst becomes implanted at a site other than the endometrial lining of the uterine cavity and the most common location is the fallopian tube.Etiology of ectopic pregnancy is unknown but risk factors includeprevious ectopic pregnancy, tubal pathology, and in-utero exposure to diethyl stilbestrol. The incidence is about 2/100 diagnosed pregnancies and ectopic pregnancy is suspected in any female of reproductive age with the early classic symptoms of abdominal pain, amenorrhea,vaginal bleeding, and unexplained syncope.Ectopic pregnancy is a gynecologic emergency and potentially life-threatening condition.Hemorrhage from ectopic pregnancy is still the leading cause of pregnancy related maternal death in

[*] Corresponding author: Chi-Wen Juan, Address: No.117, Shatian Road Shalu District, Taichung City 433, Taiwan (R.O.C.), Telephone: 886-4-26625111 ext 2001, Fax: 04-26655050, Email: juanchiwen@yahoo.com.tw

the first trimester, despite improved diagnostic methods. The diagnosis is usually made clinically, based upon the imaging studies (ultrasound) and laboratory tests (hCG). The combination of transvaginal ultrasonography and serum human chorionic gonadotrophin will allow a definitive diagnosis in almost all cases at a very early stage of pregnancy, thereby permitting treatment options.The guiding principle has become a conservative approach that attempts to save the tube, rather than salpingectomy.In the absence of emergent surgical indication, medical therapy with methotrexate is an option and its overall success rate in properly selectedwomen is significantly high.

Introduction

Ectopic pregnancy occurs when the developing blastocyst becomes implanted at a site other than the endometrium of the uterine cavity. The most common extra-uterine location is the fallopian tube, which accounts for 98 percent of all ectopic gestations . Management of these pregnancies has changed dramatically over the years [1]. The guiding principle has become a conservative approach that attempts to save the tube, rather than salpingectomy. However, it is important to remember that hemorrhage from ectopic pregnancy is still the leading cause of pregnancy related maternal death in the first trimester and accounts for 4 to 10 percent of all pregnancy related deaths, despite improved diagnostic methods leading to earlier detection and treatment [2, 3].

Incidence and Epidemiology

The prevalence of ectopic pregnancy among women who go to an emergency department with first trimester bleeding, pain, or both ranges from six to 16 percent [4]. The overall incidence of ectopic pregnancy increased during the mid twentieth century, plateauing at approximately almost 20 per 1000 pregnancies in the early 1990s, the last time national data were reported by the Centers for Disease Control [2]. This rising incidence is strongly associated with an increased incidence of pelvic inflammatory disease [5].

The current incidence of ectopic pregnancy is difficult to estimate from available data (hospitalizations, insurance billing records) because inpatient hospital treatment of ectopic pregnancy has decreased and multiple health care visits for a single ectopic pregnancy have increased [6].

Ectopic pregnancy occurs with some seasonal variation and is most common in June and December [7]. The reason is unclear.

The ectopic pregnancy maternal mortality ratio declined by 57 percent between the periods of 1980 to 1984 and 2003 to 2007, from 1.15 to 0.50 deaths per 100,000 live births [8]. The mortality ratio was 3.5 times higher for women older than 35 years than those younger than 25 years during 2003 to 2007.

Risk Factors

Risk factors for ectopic pregnancy can be divided into those that confer high, moderate, or low risk factors [4, 9, 10].

High Risk Factors

1. *Previous ectopic pregnancy* — Women who have had conservative treatment for ectopic pregnancy are at high risk (15 percent overall) for recurrence. This risk is related to both the underlying tubal disorder that led to the initial ectopic pregnancy and to the choice of treatment procedure.
2. *Tubal pathology and surgery* — The major cause of ectopic pregnancy is disruption of normal tubal anatomy from risk factors such as infection, surgery, congenital anomalies, or tumors.

- *Reconstructive surgery* — The association between tubal reconstructive surgery and subsequent ectopic pregnancy depends upon the condition of the tube, the type of surgery, and the surgeon's expertise. The tubal surgery itself is not the main cause of ectopic pregnancy; rather, the underlying tubal damage resulting from prior pelvic inflammatory disease or a prior ectopic pregnancy is the major culprit.
- *Sterilization* — The estimated failure rate during the first year after tubal sterilization ranges from 0.1 to 0.8 percent; approximately one-third of these pregnancies are ectopic. The risk of sterilization failure was illustrated by a long-term, multicenter, prospective cohort study that followed 10,685 women after tubal sterilization [11].

The major additional findings from this analysis were:

- The risk of ectopic pregnancy was higher in women sterilized before the age of 30
- Bipolar coagulation was more likely to result in ectopic pregnancy than postpartum partial salpingectomy (31.9 versus 1.2 ectopic pregnancies per 1000 procedures)
- The annual rate of ectopic pregnancy for all methods combined was similar in the first three years and in the fourth through tenth years after sterilization

3. *In-utero DES exposure* — Women with a history of in-utero diethylstilbestrol (DES) exposure have a ninefold-increased risk of ectopic pregnancy due to abnormal tubal morphology and, possibly, impaired fimbrial function [12].

Other Risk Factors

1. Previous genital infections
2. Intrauterine devices
3. Infertility
4. Multiple sexual partners
5. Smoking
6. In vitro fertilization
7. Vaginal douching
8. Age
9. Protective factors

Pathology

Almost all ectopic pregnancies occur in the fallopian tube (98 percent). In one series of 1800 surgically treated cases, the distribution of sites was ampullary (70 percent), isthmic (12 percent), fimbrial (11.1 percent), ovarian (3.2 percent), interstitial (2.4 percent), and abdominal (1.3 percent) [13].

Regardless of the location, the endometrium often responds to ovarian and placental production of pregnancy related hormones. The most common types of endometrium associated with ectopic pregnancy are decidual reaction (42 percent), secretory endometrium (22 percent), and proliferative endometrium (12 percent) [14].

Types of ectopic pregnancy:

1. *Tubal pregnancy* — As discussed above, 70 percent of tubal pregnancies occur in the ampullary portion of the fallopian tube, with the remainder about equally divided between the fimbrial and isthmus ends [15,16]. Several factors may be involved in the pathogenesis of tubal pregnancies, but they are generally believed to be the result of

    a) conditions that delay or prevent passage of the fertilized oocyte into the uterine cavity or
    b) factors inherent in the embryo that result in premature implantation.

Tubal conditions that can impair tubal transport include:

a. *Chronicsalpingitis* — Tubal pathology, particularly chronic salpingitis, is observed in up to 90 percent of ectopic pregnancies. Chronic salpingitis is six times more common in tubes containing an ectopic pregnancy than in normal tubes [17].
b. *Salpingitisisthmicanodosa* — Salpingitisisthmicanodosa (SIN) is noted in approximately 10 percent of women with a tubal pregnancy. The gross appearance of SIN is bilateral nodularities in the isthmic portion of the tube.
   A number of factors (eg, lectin, integrin, matrix-degrading cumulus, prostaglandins, growth factors, cytokines, and modular proteins) may cause premature implantation in the tube [18].

2. *Cervical pregnancy* — A cervical pregnancy is a rare form of ectopic pregnancy in which the trophoblast implants in the cervical tissue of the endocervical canal.
3. *Ovarian pregnancy* — Ovarian pregnancy occurs in 1:7000 pregnancies and is becoming more common or approximately 0.5 to 3 percent of ectopic pregnancies [19,20]. In contrast to tubal pregnancy, a history of pelvic inflammatory disease or the use of an intrauterine contraceptive device does not increase the risk of ovarian pregnancy.

Strict histopathological criteria are used to distinguish ovarian pregnancies from those originating in the fallopian tube [21].

4. *Interstitial or cornual pregnancy* — A pregnancy implanted at the interstitial portion of the fallopian tube is called an interstitial pregnancy. Originally, the term cornual pregnancy referred only to pregnancies implanted in either the horn of a bicornuate uterus, a rudimentary horn of a unicornuate uterus, or in the lateral half of a septated or partially septated uterus [22,23]. Contrary to previous belief, rupture of interstitial pregnancy occurs relatively early in pregnancy [24].
5. *Angular pregnancy* — Angular pregnancy is an intrauterine pregnancy with a clinical course distinct from interstitial pregnancy [42,43]. In contrast with an interstitial pregnancy, an angular pregnancy is located medial to the round ligament [25,26].
6. *Hysterotomy scar pregnancy* — Ectopic pregnancy in a previous hysterotomy (cesarean) scar occurs in about 1 in 2000 pregnancies and 6 percent of ectopic pregnancies among women with a prior cesarean delivery [27]. It does not appear to be related to the number of cesarean deliveries. Implantation in this location is believed to occur because the embryo migrates through a defect within the scar [28].
7. *Heterotopic pregnancy* — Heterotopic pregnancy refers to the combination of an intrauterine pregnancy and a concurrent pregnancy at an ectopic location. The incidence has been rising, mainly due to the increasing number of pregnancies derived from assisted reproductive technology (ART). A few cases have been diagnosed as late as 16 weeks of gestation.
8. *Abdominal pregnancy* — An abdominal pregnancy may be primary, from direct implantation of the blastocyst on the peritoneal surface or abdominal viscera, or secondary, resulting from extrusion of an embryo from the tube [29]. In a review of deliveries over a 20 year period at one institution, the incidence of abdominal pregnancy was approximately 1:5000 deliveries with nine early and six advanced abdominal gestations [30].

Clinical Manifestations

Clinical manifestations typically appear six to eight weeks after the last normal menstrual period, but can occur later, especially if the pregnancy is not in the fallopian tube. Normal pregnancy discomforts (eg, breast tenderness, frequent urination, nausea) are often present in addition to the symptoms described below.

History — The classic symptoms of ectopic pregnancy are [31]:

- Abdominal pain
- Amenorrhea
- Vaginal bleeding

These symptoms can occur in both ruptured and unruptured cases. Abdominal pain was a presenting symptom in 99 percent, amenorrhea in 74 percent, and vaginal bleeding in 56 percent [32]

Ectopic pregnancy should be suspected in any women of reproductive age with these symptoms, especially those who have risk factors for an extrauterine pregnancy.[33]

However, these symptoms are not diagnostic of ectopic pregnancy; they are the same as those associated with threatened abortion, which is far more common.

In addition, blood leaking out of the fallopian tube may irritate the diaphragm and cause shoulder pain.

A population-based French study identified four factors that increased the risk of rupture when an ectopic pregnancy was suspected:

(1) never having used contraception
(2) history of tubal damage and infertility,
(3) induction of ovulation, and
(4) high level of human chorionic gonadotropin (at least 10,000 IU/L) [34].

Physical examination — Vital signs may reveal orthostatic changes and, occasionally, low grade fever. Findings on physical examination may include adnexal, cervical motion, and/or abdominal tenderness, an adnexal mass, and mild uterine enlargement.

However, the physical examination is often unremarkable in a woman with a small, unruptured ectopic pregnancy.

Laboratory Evaluation

Complete blood count, Blood type and screen — Women with ectopic pregnancy should be evaluated for anemia, platelets and coagulation tests.

Diagnosis

No constellation of historical and physical findings can confirm or exclude the diagnosis of ectopic pregnancy with a high degree of reliability. [35,36]. The diagnosis is usually made clinically, based upon results of the imaging studies (ultrasound) and laboratory tests (hCG) described below.

Differential diagnosis — The differential diagnosis of lower abdominal pain in women includes urinary tract infection, appendicitis, ovarian neoplasms, endometriosis, endometritis, leiomyomas, pelvic inflammatory disease, and pregnancy-related conditions.

Vaginal bleeding also has several pregnancy-related and nonpregnancy-related etiologies. Thus, a pregnancy test is important in premenopausal women who present with abdominal pain or vaginal bleeding in order to guide the direction of further evaluation.

Recommended diagnostic tests — TVUS is the most useful test for determining the location of a pregnancy. If the imaging study is nondiagnostic, it may be because the gestation is too early to be visualized on ultrasound. If so, serial measurements of the serum human chorionic gonadotropin (hCG) concentration should be taken until the hCG discriminatory zone is reached.

This combination of TVUS and hCG will permit a definitive diagnosis in almost all cases at a very early stage of pregnancy, thereby permitting treatment options less invasive than surgical excision [37-40].

Transvaginal ultrasound (TVUS) — Ultrasound is used to detect the presence (or absence) of a pregnancy within or outside of the uterus. Ultrasound evaluation for ectopic pregnancy is discussed in detail separately.

Human chorionic gonadotropin — Measurement of serum hCG is performed to diagnose pregnancy and then repeated serially (typically every two days) to assess whether the increase in concentration is consistent with an abnormal pregnancy. In some cases, the diagnosis of ectopic pregnancy can be made after a single measurement of hCG, if pelvic ultrasound findings suggest an ectopic pregnancy.

The hCG concentration in a normal intrauterine pregnancy rises in a curvilinear fashion until about 41 days of gestation, after which it rises more slowly until approximately 10 weeks, and then declines until reaching a plateau in the second and third trimesters [41-43].

Studies in viable intrauterine pregnancies have reported the following changes in serum hCG [44-48]:

The hCG concentration rises at a much slower rate in most, but not all, ectopic and nonviable intrauterine pregnancies [49,50]. There is a 10 to 15 percent interassay variability in hCG measurements as well as variability among laboratories. Thus, interpretation of serial hCG concentrations is more reliable when the assays are performed in the same laboratory. In addition, the possibility of falsely positive hCG test results should be considered [51-54]. A falling hCG concentration is most consistent with a failed pregnancy.

Discriminatory zone — The discriminatory zone is based upon the correlation between visibility of the gestational sac and the hCG concentration, and is of major diagnostic importance It is defined as the serum hCG level above which a gestational sac should be visualized by ultrasound examination if an intrauterine pregnancy is present.

The level of the discriminatory zone was based upon observations that an intrauterine gestational sac could be detected by TVUS in patients with serum hCG concentrations as low as 800 IU/L and was usually identified by expert ultrasonographers at concentrations above 1500 to 2000 IU/L [55]. In one representative study, 185 of 188 (98 percent) intrauterine pregnancies in women with hCG above 1500 IU/L were visualized [56].

The absence of an intrauterine gestational sac at hCG concentrations above the discriminatory zone strongly suggests an ectopic or nonviable intrauterine pregnancy, but is nondiagnostic with hCG values below the discriminatory zone.

Diagnostic evaluation — The evaluation of a pregnant woman with suspected ectopic gestation begins with TVUS and quantitative hCGlevel .

TVUS alone is diagnostic if a yolk sac, embryo, or embryonic cardiac activity is demonstrable.

HCG above the discriminatory zone — A hCG concentration above the discriminatory zone is sensitive for detecting an intrauterine pregnancy. Visualization of an intrauterine pregnancy almost always excludes the presence of an ectopic pregnancy; exceptions include heterotopic pregnancies .

If TVUS does not reveal an intrauterine pregnancy and shows a complex adnexal mass, an extrauterine pregnancy is almost certain. Embryonic cardiac activity or a gestational sac with a definite yolk sac or embryo at an extrauterine location is certain evidence of an ectopic gestation. Treatment of ectopic pregnancy should be instituted.

HCG below the discriminatory zone — TVUS is not sensitive for determining the location of the pregnancy when the hCG level is below the discriminatory zone. A serum hCG concentration less than 1500 IU/L should be followed by repetition of hCG in three days to follow the rate of rise. HCG concentrations usually double every 1.4 to two days until six to seven weeks of gestation in viable intrauterine pregnancies (and in some ectopic gestations) Measurement every 72 hours is more practical than every 48 hours.

If an adnexal mass is visualized on TVUS, then medical or surgical treatment is administered for a presumed ectopic pregnancy. If an adnexal mass is not visualized, some clinicians administer methotrexate and others perform curettage to determine the type of nonviable pregnancy and thereby avoid medical therapy of nonviable intrauterine pregnancies [57].

Ancillary Diagnostic Tests

Progesterone — Serum progesterone concentrations are higher in viable intrauterine pregnancies than in ectopic pregnancies and intrauterine pregnancies that are destined to abort [58].

The sensitivity and specificity of a low serum progesterone concentration for predicting a nonviable pregnancy in spontaneously pregnant patients are different from those in infertile patients who have undergone controlled ovarian hyperstimulation for in vitro fertilization or intrauterine insemination [59].

Curettage — The intrauterine location of a pregnancy is diagnosed with certainty if trophoblastic tissue is obtained by uterine curettage. Obviously, the use of curettage as a diagnostic tool is limited by the potential for disruption of a viable pregnancy [58].

Moreover, false negatives can occur: chorionic villi are not detected by histopathology in 20 percent of curettage specimens from elective termination of pregnancy [60]. Pipelle endometrial biopsy is even less sensitive than curettage for detection of villi; sensitivities reported in two small series were 30 and 60 percent. When an intrauterine pregnancy has been evacuated, hCG levels should drop by at least 15 percent the day after evacuation

Some authors have recommended performing curettage only on women with both a hCG concentration below the discriminatory zone and a low doubling rate

A decision analysis comparing the cost/complication rates in patients who undergo diagnostic curettage before administration of methotrexate to those who do not have a curettage concluded there was no significant benefit of one approach over the other [61]. It is more practical and less invasive to continue observation or administer one dose of methotrexate than to perform curettage [62,63].

Doppler — Blood flow in the arteries of the fallopian tube containing an ectopic pregnancy is 20 to 45 percent higher than in the opposite tube and the Doppler waveform shows low impedance [64]. Doppler support the diagnosis of ectopic pregnancy, especially if a complex adnexal mass is also visualized. In one study, the resistive index of ectopic pregnancies was higher than that of corpus luteum cyst [65]. The use of TVUS and hCG measurements is usually sufficient in establishing the diagnosis in routine clinical practice.

Laparoscopy — Laparoscopy is rarely required for diagnostic purposes only; transvaginal ultrasound examination and hCG measurements are usually sufficient for diagnosis.

Magnetic resonance imaging — Magnetic resonance imaging can be used to diagnose ectopic pregnancy, but is a cost effective approach [66].

SCREENING ASYMPTOMATIC WOMEN — Over 50 percent of women are asymptomatic before tubal rupture and do not have an identifiable risk factor for ectopic pregnancy [67].

A decision analysis model showed that screening asymptomatic pregnant women for ectopic pregnancy reduced the frequency of rupture, but approximately three false positive diagnoses would occur per tubal rupture prevented if the prevalence of ectopic pregnancy was 2 percent [68].

UNCOMMON TYPES OF ECTOPIC PREGNANCY — The possibility that an ectopic pregnancy may occur in a nontubal location, in conjunction with an intrauterine pregnancy, or even bilaterally [69], should be considered. Regardless of the location, the endometrium often responds to ovarian and placental production of pregnancy related hormones, so vaginal bleeding is a common symptom.

- Cervical pregnancy is estimated to occur in 1/2500 to 1/18,000 pregnancies and accounts for 1 percent of ectopic pregnancies [70-72].
- Ovarian pregnancy occurs in 1/2100 to 1/60,000 pregnancies and accounts for 1 to 3 percent of ectopic pregnancies [73].
- Interstitial pregnancy accounts for up to 1 to 3 percent of ectopic pregnancies [74, 75].
- Abdominal pregnancy accounts for up to 1.4 percent of ectopic pregnancies [76-78]. These pregnancies can go undetected until an advanced age and often result in severe hemorrhage [79]. Rates of maternal mortality have been reported as high as 20 percent [80,81].
- Intramural pregnancy refers to pregnancy implanted within the myometrium of the uterus. This type of pregnancy is extremely rare with less than 50 reported cases in the literature [82].

Heterotopic pregnancy — Early diagnosis of heterotopic pregnancy is difficult because of lack of symptoms. On ultrasound examination, the diagnosis is suggested by visualization of both an ectopic and intrauterine pregnancy or the presence of echogenic fluid in the posterior cul de sac in the presence of an intrauterine pregnancy. Heterotopic tubal pregnancies have been reported as late as 16 weeks of gestation, while abdominal or rudimentary horn pregnancies can continue to develop late in gestation [83]

Women with a confirmed intrauterine pregnancy who are experiencing abdominal or pelvic pain undergo serial TVS examinations every week until the possibility of a concomitant tubal ectopic pregnancy can be eliminated.

If the ectopic pregnancy has not ruptured, then local injection of 5 mEq potassium chloride into the sac is another option [84-88].

Cervical pregnancy — The most common symptom of cervical pregnancy is vaginal bleeding, which is often profuse and painless. Lower abdominal pain or cramps occur in fewer than one-third of patients; pain without bleeding is rare. Diagnosis and management of cervical pregnancy are discussed in detail separately.

Hysterotomy scar pregnancy — Symptoms are similar to tubal ectopic pregnancy, and include vaginal bleeding and abdominal pain. The diagnosis is made by sonographically visualizing an enlarged hysterotomy scar with an embedded mass [89] Features which should be present include presence of trophoblast between the bladder and the anterior uterine wall, no fetal parts in the uterine cavity, absence of myometrium between the gestational sac and the bladder, and Doppler evidence of perfusion of the peritrophoblastic vasculature [89-91].

If the pregnancy has not ruptured, then local injection of potassium chloride into the sac under sonographic guidance is an effective treatment. Rupture can result in significant bleeding

Ovarian pregnancy — Sonographic diagnosis of an ovarian pregnancy is difficult. The diagnosis of ovarian pregnancy is typically made at the time of surgery, but differentiation from a hemorrhagic ovarian cyst or pregnancy in the distal fallopian tube can be difficult. Ultrasound may suggest the diagnosis preoperatively [45]. Strict histopathological criteria are used to distinguish ovarian pregnancies from those originating in the fallopian tube. The exact diagnosis is not clinically important as these pregnancies are usually treated by surgical excision of the involved organs. Methotrexate treatment has been successful in case reports [92-95].

Abdominal pregnancy — Abdominal pregnancy is associated with a wide range of signs and symptoms. These include abdominal pain, vaginal bleeding, vomiting, painful fetal movement, oligohydramnios, persistent unusual fetal lie, failure to deliver an intrauterine fetal demise, and labor abnormalities. In one report, hemothorax developed from implantation on the diaphragm [96].

Interstitial pregnancy — A pregnancy implanted at the interstitial portion of the fallopian tube is called an interstitial pregnancy. Originally, the term cornual pregnancy referred only to pregnancies implanted in either the horn of a bicornuate uterus, a rudimentary horn of a unicornuate uterus, or in one side of a septated or partially septated uterus [97].

Grossly, an interstitial pregnancy appears as a gestational swelling lateral to the insertion of the round ligament [98]. An average delay in diagnosis of only four days in comparison with tubal pregnancies was reported in a large series [98].

Interstitial pregnancy presents with rupture in approximately 20 to 50 percent of cases [99- 101]. A series of cases of interstitial pregnancy reported to a surgical registry included 14 patients with tubal rupture, all of which were before 12 weeks [99]. Other clinical manifestations are the same as for all ectopic gestations (pelvic or abdominal pain, vaginal bleeding) [98].

NATURAL HISTORY — If left untreated, an ectopic pregnancy in the fallopian tube can progress to a tubal abortion or tubal rupture, or it may regress spontaneously.

- Spontaneous resolution — The incidence of spontaneous resolution of an ectopic pregnancy is unknown. In one older (1955) series of 119 hospitalized patients with typical ectopic pregnancy symptoms, 57 were safely managed expectantly, without surgical or medical intervention (except opiates) [102]. It is difficult to predict which patients will experience uncomplicated spontaneous resolution. Potential candidates are hemodynamically stable women with an initial hCG concentration less than 2000 IU/L that is declining [103-105]. Gestational products left in the fallopian tube may resorb completely or, less commonly, may cause tubal obstruction [106]. Alternatively, a tubal abortion may occur.

Expectant Management of Ectopic Pregnancy

Ectopic pregnancy is a gynecologic emergency, generally requiring expeditious surgical or medical treatment. However, in a small number of cases in which the risk of tubal rupture is minimal, expectant management is appropriate. Women who are candidates for expectant management of ectopic pregnancy require informed consent about the risks of this strategy and close observation until the pregnancy has resolved.

In a historic study, expectant management versus surgery in women with ectopic pregnancy, regardless of risk factors for tubal rupture, resulted in a 57 percent success rate [107]. However, most of the patients who failed this approach had significant complications (i.e., tubal rupture) or ultimately required surgery for ongoing pregnancy.

The use of more stringent selection criteria results in an increase in the efficacy of expectant management to approximately 70 percent [108]. Success rates vary from 48 to 100 percent, depending in large part on differences in inclusion criteria [109].

Candidates for Expectant Management

Selection criteria — When ectopic pregnancy is suspected, expectant management are employed only for patients who meet the following criteria:

(1) transvaginal ultrasound (TVUS) does not show a gestational sac or demonstrate an extrauterine mass suspicious for an ectopic pregnancy and
(2) the beta-human chorionic gonadotropin (hCG) concentration is low (<200 mIU/mL) and declining [110]. This also the threshold advised by the American College of Obstetricians and Gynecologists (ACOG) [111].

A declining hCG level is defined as lower at the third measurement than at the first measurement.

Patients with no extrauterine mass on TVUS can be described as a pregnancy of unknown location since imaging and laboratory assessment do not clearly distinguish between a failed intrauterine pregnancy and a resolving ectopic pregnancy at this low level of hCG. An extrauterine mass could represent an involuting ectopic pregnancy or another type of adnexal mass.

If expectant management is offered, the patient must be aware of and accept the risks and be willing and able to comply with follow-up. As with all patients managed expectantly, such women should be treated medically or surgically if hCG levels are increasing or if there are signs of tubal rupture. We do not perform endometrial sampling in the management of ectopic pregnancy.

The upper limit of serum hCG level that allows for expectant management of ectopic pregnancy without unnecessary risk of tubal rupture is unknown. Several studies have evaluated use of ahCG threshold higher than 200 mIU/mL [110,112,113]. This was best evaluated in a randomized trial (n = 73) that assigned women with an ectopic pregnancy or pregnancy of unknown location (PUL) and a plateauing hCG level to methotrexate (MTX) therapy or expectant management [113]. The hCG cutoffs were <1500 mIU/mL for ectopic pregnancy or <2000 mIU/mL for PUL. The initial treatment was sufficient more often in women treated with MTX than expectant management (76 versus 39 percent), but this did not reach statistical significance (relative risk 1.3, 95% CI 0.9-1.8). In the expectant management group, 28 percent of women were subsequently treated with MTX. Surgery was required in 1 of 41 women (2 percent) in the MTX group and 4 of 32 (13 percent) in the expectant management group.

In the trial cited above, a large proportion of patients assigned to expectant management ultimately required MTX and more patients required surgery, although the risk of surgery is based on few events [113]. Taking into account the potentially serious risks of tubal rupture and hemorrhage with ectopic pregnancy and the safety and efficacy of medical and surgical treatment, we recommend that the more stringent hCG criterion (>200 mIU/mL) should be used for expectant management. Further study, particularly of hCG thresholds between 200 and 1500 mIU/mL, is warranted.

Contraindications — Expectant treatment should not be attempted or should be abandoned in women with known or suspected ectopic pregnancy with the following characteristics:

- Hemodynamically unstable
- Signs of impending or ongoing ectopic mass rupture (i.e., severe or persistent abdominal pain or >300 mL of free peritoneal fluid outside the pelvic cavity)
- hCG that is greater than 200 mIU/mL, is increasing, or is not declining
- Unwilling or unable to comply with monitoring
- Does not have timely access to a medical institution

OUTCOME — Success rates for expectant management of ectopic pregnancy of 48 to 100 percent have been reported. The wide variation is due, in part, to differences in inclusion criteria [108-110,114,115]. Expectant management appears reasonable in selected patients based upon the following data:

FOLLOW-UP — Patients treated with expectant management should be monitored closely. Tubal rupture has been reported in women with low and declining hCG levels.

Following of the hCG level is suggested every 48 hours for three measurements to confirm that it continues to decline, and then weekly until it is undetectable, at which point tubal rupture is highly unlikely. Asymptomatic women who are managed expectantly and have hCG levels that are slowly declining or have plateaued can be offered continuation of expectant management or methotrexate injection.

Expectant treatment should be abandoned if a patient experiences significant increase in abdominal pain, serum hCG starts to increase or fails to decrease, or a patient experiences increasing abdominal pain.

Methotrexate Treatment of Tubal and Interstitial Ectopic Pregnancy

Ectopic pregnancy is a potentially life-threatening condition. While surgical approaches are the mainstay of treatment, advances in early diagnosis facilitated the introduction of medical therapy with methotrexate (MTX) in the 1980s [116]. In one report, approximately 35 percent of women with ectopic pregnancy are eligible for medical treatment [117]. The overall success rate of medical treatment in properly selected women is nearly 90 percent [118-120].

PHARMACOLOGY — MTX is a folic acid antagonist widely used for treatment of neoplasia, severe psoriasis, and rheumatoid arthritis.

MTX is rapidly cleared from the body by the kidneys, with 90 percent of an intravenous (IV) dose excreted unchanged within 24 hours of administration [121].

The dose of MTX used to treat ectopic pregnancy (50 mg/m2 or 1 mg/kg) is relatively low. High dose MTX (>500 mg/m2) is used to treat some malignancies.In some protocols, reduced folates (leucovorin, also called folinic acid, N5-formyl-tetrahydrofolate, citrovorum factor) are given to bypass the metabolic block induced by MTX, and thus rescue normal cells from toxicity. Preliminary research has been done to investigate use of a combination of MTX and gefitinib, a medication used in the treatment of non–small cell lung cancer and breast cancer [122-123].

Candidates for Medical Treatment

Optimal candidates — The optimal candidates for MTX treatment of ectopic pregnancy are hemodynamically stable, willing and able to comply with posttreatment follow-up, have a human chorionic gonadotropin beta-subunit (hCG) concentration <5000 mIU/mL, and no fetal cardiac activity.

Contraindications — Some women are not appropriate candidates for medical therapy and should be managed surgically, including women with the following characteristics [124-125]:

- Hemodynamically unstable
- Signs of impending or ongoing ectopic mass rupture (i.e., severe or persistent abdominal pain or >300 mL of free peritoneal fluid outside the pelvic cavity)
- Clinically important abnormalities in baseline hematologic, renal or hepatic laboratory values
- Immunodeficiency, active pulmonary disease, peptic ulcer disease
- Hypersensitivity to MTX
- Coexistent viable intrauterine pregnancy
- Breastfeeding
- Unwilling or unable to be compliant with post-therapeutic monitoring
- Do not have timely access to a medical institution

MTX is renally cleared, and in women with renal insufficiency, a single dose of MTX can lead to death or severe complications. Dialysis does not provide normal renal clearance [126 ,127].

Relative Contraindications

- High hCG concentration
- Fetal cardiac activity
- Large ectopic size — Large size of the ectopic pregnancy (>3.5 cm) is often used as criterion for exclusion in medical treatment regimens, this restriction is based on small studies with inconsistent protocols and results [128-131].
- Peritoneal fluid

DRUG ADMINISTRATION — MTX can be given systemically (intravenously, intramuscularly, or orally) or by direct local injection into the ectopic pregnancy sac transvaginally or laparoscopically. Intramuscular (IM) administration is most common.

Efficacy of single versus multidose therapy — The two most commonly used protocols for MTX administration are single dose and multiple dose (four MTX doses which alternate with oral leucovorin).

Multiple dose protocols appear to cause more adverse effects [118]. The single dose approach is less expensive, requires less intensive monitoring, and does not require folinic acid rescue.

Combination therapy with mifepristone —A systematic review of randomized trials of single dose intramuscular MTX (50 mg/m2) in combination with oral mifepristone (600 mg) versus MTX alone found that combination therapy may increase treatment efficacy. Success rates for MTX or MTX/mifepristone therapy were 81 and 74 percent; the difference approached statistical significance.

Pretreatment testing — Prior to treatment, a viable pregnancy must be excluded. Otherwise, a woman with an intrauterine pregnancy might be subjected to methotrexate administration [132].

The following testing should be performed:

- Serum hCG as part of the diagnostic evaluation and to establish a baseline to monitor the effect of therapy
- Transvaginal ultrasound as part of the diagnostic evaluation
- Blood type and screen to determine the need for anti-D immune globulin in women who are Rh(D)-negative
- Complete blood count and renal and liver function tests to assess for contraindications to MTX therapy.

Precautions during Therapy

- Avoid vaginal intercourse and new conception until hCG is undetectable
- Avoid pelvic exams during surveillance of MTX therapy due to theoretical risk of tubal rupture

- Avoid sun exposure to limit risk of MTX dermatitis
- Avoid foods and vitamins containing folic acid
- Avoid nonsteroidalantiinflammatory drugs

Single dose protocol — The most efficient approach to medical therapy is administration of a single IM dose of MTX. Approximately 15 to 20 percent of women will require a second dose of MTX and patients should be made aware of this before starting the protocol [118,129] Fewer than 1 percent of patients need more than two doses [118].

In the single dose protocol, Day 1 is the day that MTX is administered [118,133] The dose used is 50 mg per square meter of body surface area (BSA) [134].

Posttreatment Management

Ultrasound follow-up — After treatment, the ectopic pregnancy is often noted to increase in size and may persist for weeks on serial ultrasound examinations.

Side effects and complications — Adverse reactions to MTX are usually mild and self-limited. The most common are stomatitis and conjunctivitis.

Pain after treatment — Mild abdominal pain of short duration (one to two days) six to seven days after receiving the medication is also common. The pain may be due to tubal abortion or tubal distention from hematoma formation and can usually be controlled with acetaminophen.

Women with severe pain should be closely observed for hemodynamic changes which may accompany a tubal rupture.

Subsequent Reproductive Performance

Interval to conception — One study reported that patients with ectopic pregnancies treated with MTX had a timely return of menses and superior rates of conception compared with those treated with conservative surgical management [135].

Toxicology literature recommends a four to six month washout period [185-186].

Effect on fertility — There is no evidence of adverse effects of MTX treatment of ectopic pregnancy on future pregnancies [136-139]. In addition, treatment with MTX does not appear to compromise ovarian reserve [140]. Attempts to conceive may be resumed after the hCG level is undetectable. In a study of women treated with in vitro fertilization, ovarian responses among women with a history of ectopic pregnancy treated with methotrexate or salpingectomy were comparable [141].

The incidence of recurrent ectopic pregnancy is approximately 15 percent and rises to 30 percent following two ectopic pregnancies [142]. The risk of recurrence appears to be the same for both medical and surgical therapies [143].

The initial level of hCG>5000 mIU/mL may be associated with increased risk of subsequent tubal obstruction, regardless of treatment approach [144].

Surgical Treatment of Ectopic Pregnancy

Management of ectopic pregnancy has dramatically moved away from a primarily surgical approach [145]. Currently, most women with unruptured ectopic pregnancies are treated with methotrexate. However, some women undergo surgical therapy by choice or by necessity, if they are not good candidates for medical therapy.

Indications for Surgical Treatment

- Hemodynamic instability
- Impending or ongoing rupture of ectopic mass
- Contraindications to methotrexate
- Coexisting intrauterine pregnancy
- Not able or willing to comply with medical therapy post-treatment follow-up
- Lack of timely access to a medical institution for management of tubal rupture
- Desire for permanent contraception

- Known tubal disease with planned in vitro fertilization for future pregnancy (only in patients who are otherwise good candidates for surgical therapy)
- Failed medical therapy

In addition, women with a serum beta human chorionic gonadotropin (hCG) concentration greater than 5000 mIU/mL before treatment or fetal cardiac activity on ultrasonographic examination are more likely to experience treatment failure with methotrexate treatment.

Surgical Procedure

Salpingostomy versus salpingectomy — The choice of salpingostomy or salpingectomy for treatment of ectopic pregnancy is controversial.

A review of cohort studies comparing fertility outcome after salpingostomy and salpingectomy for tubal ectopic pregnancy did not find an overall beneficial effect of salpingostomy [146]. The rate of future intrauterine pregnancy was not consistently higher after salpingostomy than after salpingectomy [145-153], whereas the risk of repeat ectopic pregnancy was slightly increased [146].

Salpingostomy is performed in women who are hemodynamically stable and appear to have a reasonable probability of future normal tubal function in the affected tube. Salpingectomy is performed in the following situations:

- Uncontrolled bleeding from the implantation site
- Recurrent ectopic pregnancy in the same tube
- Severely damaged tube
- Large tubal pregnancy (i.e., greater than 5 cm)
- Women who have completed childbearing (with or without a tubal sterilization procedure), or who will be treated with in vitro fertilization

Laparoscopy versus laparotomy — Laparoscopic surgery is the standard surgical approach for ectopic pregnancy. Laparoscopic salpingostomy resulted in significantly shorter operation time (73 versus 88 minutes), less perioperative blood loss (79 versus 195 ml), shorter duration of hospital stay

(1 to 2 versus 3 to 5 days), shorter convalescence time (11 versus 24 days), and, therefore, lower costs.

Laparoscopic salpingostomy also resulted in a higher rate of persistent trophoblast than salpingostomy via laparotomy [146].

Use of single port laparoscopy (also referred to as laparoendoscopic single-site surgery [LESS]) for ectopic pregnancy is alternative choice[154 - 157].

The only comparative study to-date reported that women with a tubal pregnancy who underwent salpingectomy with LESS compared with conventional laparoscopy had similar outcomes for operative duration, blood loss, and hospital stay [158].

Procedure for laparoscopic salpingostomy — Linear salpingostomy is the standard approach for management of ectopic pregnancy in women who wish to preserve their fertility. The ectopic pregnancy is identified and the tube is immobilized with laparoscopic forceps [159].

The incision is left open to heal by secondary intention; the subsequent rates of fertility and adhesion formation are similar after secondary intention or primary closure [160-161].

Procedure for laparoscopic salpingectomy — There are several methods for laparoscopic salpingectomy. One approach is to bring the fallopian tube through a pre-tied surgical loop using a grasping forceps . The knot is tightened and a second loop is similarly placed. The tube can then be resected and removed.

Cornuostomy or cornual resection of interstitial pregnancy — Historically, cornual resection and hysterectomy were the most common procedures for treatment of interstitial pregnancy, probably as a result of delayed diagnosis [162-165]. More recently, widespread use and availability of transvaginal ultrasound and sensitive beta-hCG assays has allowed diagnosis of these pregnancies at an earlier gestational age and prior to rupture, thus providing an opportunity for conservative medical or surgical treatment [166].

These patients are initially treated medically [162,166-168], resorting to surgical therapy if there is any deterioration in clinical status. Laparoscopic removal of the gestation via cornuostomy, with resection of the interstitial portion of the tube (cornual resection) is preferred if necessary. [169].

Successful hysteroscopic removal of interstitial ectopic pregnancy has been described [170,171]. The efficacy and long-term results of this technique are unknown.

Unfortunately, the risk of uterine rupture after medical treatment of an interstitial pregnancy is unknown and the integrity of the uterus following conservative surgical treatment is unclear, although cases of uterine rupture have been reported [171-173].

Outcome and Prognosis

Persistent ectopic pregnancy — The incidence of persistent ectopic pregnancy reported in case series ranges from 4 to 15 percent, and, as noted above, is generally higher after laparoscopic salpingostomy than after open procedures [174].

The clearance rate of serum beta-hCG following salpingostomy is similar to that after salpingectomy. One study found that the serum beta-hCG concentration on the first postoperative day generally declined by more than 50 percent of the preoperative value. In this series of 147 women treated conservatively for ectopic pregnancy, there were no cases of persistent ectopic pregnancy when the postoperative beta-hCG on day 1 fell by more than 76 percent [175].

Alternatively, prophylactic treatment with one dose of methotrexate can be given after all salpingostomies [176].

The pregnancy rate was comparable to that in women who were successfully treated for their primary ectopic pregnancy [177].

Future pregnancy — Ectopic implantation usually occurs because clinical or subclinical salpingitis has caused anatomic and functional changes in the fallopian tubes. These changes are typically bilateral and permanent; thus, it is not surprising that ectopic pregnancy often leads to recurrent ectopic pregnancy and infertility.

- *Recurrent ectopic pregnancy* — The incidence of recurrent ectopic pregnancy is approximately 15 percent (range 4 to 28 percent) [31].After methotrexate treatment, the recurrent ectopic rates range between 10.2 percent to 18.7 percent [178,179]. The differences could be related to the varied condition of the fallopian tubes. The recurrence risk rises to 30 percent following two ectopic pregnancies

[180]. As an example, a prospective study followed 328 women who were not using intrauterine contraception at the time of their ectopic pregnancy, and who subsequently tried to become pregnant [178].

- A history of prior infertility is the most important factor for predicting subsequent fertility [181]. The pregnancy rate following ectopic pregnancy in women with a history of infertility is one-fourth that of women without known infertility [182].
- Ipsilateralperiadnexal adhesions reflect poor condition of the tube [183].
- Among 23 intrauterine contraception users, there was no recurrence of ectopic pregnancy, while 28 percent of 305 nonusers had recurrences in the following two years [184].

Almost all (93 percent) spontaneous pregnancies after surgical treatment of ectopic pregnancy occur in the first 18 months following the procedure [185].

Interval to conception — There are no data to establish the optimal interval to conception following surgical treatment of an ectopic pregnancy.

References

[1] Yao M, Tulandi T. Current status of surgical and nonsurgical management of ectopic pregnancy. *FertilSteril.,* 1997; 67:421.

[2] Centers for Disease Control and Prevention (CDC). Ectopic pregnancy--United States, 1990-1992. *MMWR Morb. Mortal. Wkly. Rep.,* 1995; 44:46.

[3] Fylstra DL. Tubal pregnancy: a review of current diagnosis and treatment. *Obstet. Gynecol. Surv.,* 1998; 53:320.

[4] Murray H, Baakdah H, Bardell T, Tulandi T. Diagnosis and treatment of ectopic pregnancy. *CMAJ,* 2005; 173:905.

[5] Kamwendo F, Forslin L, Bodin L, Danielsson D. Epidemiology of ectopic pregnancy during a 28 year period and the role of pelvic inflammatory disease. *Sex Transm. Infect.,* 2000; 76:28.

[6] Zane SB, Kieke BA Jr, Kendrick JS, Bruce C. Surveillance in a time of changing health care practices: estimating ectopic pregnancy incidence in the United States. *Matern. Child Health J.,* 2002; 6:227.

[7] Cagnacci A, Landi S, Volpe A. Rhythmic variation in the rate of ectopic pregnancy throughout the year. *Am. J. Obstet. Gynecol.,* 1999; 180:1067.

[8] Creanga AA, Shapiro-Mendoza CK, Bish CL, et al. Trends in ectopic pregnancy mortality in the United States: 1980-2007. *Obstet. Gynecol.,* 2011; 117:837.

[9] Ankum WM, Mol BW, Van der Veen F, Bossuyt PM. Risk factors for ectopic pregnancy: a meta-analysis. *Fertil. Steril.,* 1996; 65:1093.

[10] Bouyer J, Coste J, Shojaei T, et al. Risk factors for ectopic pregnancy: a comprehensive analysis based on a large case-control, population-based study in France. *Am. J. Epidemiol.,* 2003; 157:185.

[11] Peterson HB, Xia Z, Hughes JM, et al. The risk of ectopic pregnancy after tubal sterilization.U.S. Collaborative Review of Sterilization Working Group. *N. Engl. J. Med.,* 1997; 336:762.

[12] Goldberg JM, Falcone T. Effect of diethylstilbestrol on reproductive function. *Fertil. Steril.,* 1999; 72.

[13] Bouyer J, Coste J, Fernandez H, et al. Sites of ectopic pregnancy: a 10 year population-based study of 1800 cases. *Hum. Reprod.,* 2002; 17:32 24.

[14] Lopez HB, Micheelsen U, Berendtsen H, Kock K. Ectopic pregnancy and its associated endometrial changes. *Gynecol. Obstet. Invest.,* 1994; 38:104.

[15] Senterman M, Jibodh R, Tulandi T. Histopathologic study of ampullary and isthmic tubal ectopic pregnancy. *Am. J. Obstet. Gynecol.,* 1988; 159: 939.

[16] Kutluay L, Vicdan K, Turan C, et al. Tubal histopathology in ectopic pregnancies. *Eur. J. Obstet. Gynecol. Reprod. Biol.,* 1994; 57:91.

[17] Attar E. Endocrinology of ectopic pregnancy. *Obstet. Gynecol. Clin. North Am., 2004*; 31:779.

[18] Gaudoin MR, Coulter KL, Robins AM, et al. Is the incidence of ovarian ectopic pregnancy increasing? *Eur. J. Obstet. Gynecol. Reprod. Biol.,* 1996; 70:141.

[19] Raziel A, Golan A, Pansky M, et al. Ovarian pregnancy: a report of twenty cases in one institution. *Am. J. Obstet. Gynecol.,* 1990; 163:1182.

[20] Spiegelberg, O. Zurcasvistik des ovarialsschwangerschaft. *Arch. Gynack.,* 1878; 13:73.

[21] Lau S, Tulandi T. Conservative medical and surgical management of interstitial ectopic pregnancy. *Fertil. Steril.,* 1999; 72:207.

[22] Jansen RP, Elliott PM. Angular intrauterine pregnancy. *Obstet. Gynecol.,* 1981; 58:167.

[23] Tulandi T, Al-Jaroudi D. Interstitial pregnancy: results generated from the Society of Reproductive Surgeons Registry. *Obstet. Gynecol.,* 2004; 103:47.

[24] Larraín D, Marengo F, Bourdel N, et al. Proximal ectopic pregnancy: a descriptive general population-based study and results of different management options in 86 cases. *Fertil. Steril.,* 2011; 95:867.

[25] Ps B, Hk C. Angular ectopic pregnancy presenting as rupture of lateral wall of the uterus. *J. Hum. Reprod. Sci.,* 2008; 1:33.

[26] Rotas MA, Haberman S, Levgur M. Cesarean scar ectopic pregnancies: etiology, diagnosis, and management. *Obstet. Gynecol.,* 2006; 107:1373.

[27] Ash A, Smith A, Maxwell D. Caesarean scar pregnancy. *BJOG,* 2007; 114:253.

[28] Hassiakos D, Bakas P, Pistofidis G, Creatsas G. Heterotopic pregnancy at 16 weeks of gestation after in-vitro fertilization and embryo transfer. *Arch. Gynecol. Obstet.,* 2002; 266:124.

[29] Strafford JC, Ragan WD. Abdominal pregnancy. Review of current management. *Obstet. Gynecol.,* 1977; 50:548.

[30] Martin JN Jr, Sessums JK, Martin RW, et al. Abdominal pregnancy: current concepts of management. *Obstet. Gynecol.,* 1988; 71:549.

[31] 2 Ankum WM, Mol BW, Van der Veen F, Bossuyt PM. Risk factors for ectopic pregnancy: a meta-analysis. *Fertil. Steril.,* 1996; 65:1093.

[32] Alsuleiman SA, Grimes EM. Ectopic pregnancy: a review of 147 cases. *J. Reprod. Med.,* 1982; 27:101.

[33] Weckstein LN. Current perspective on ectopic pregnancy. *Obstet. Gynecol. Surv.,* 1985; 40:259.

[34] Job-Spira N, Fernandez H, Bouyer J, et al. Ruptured tubal ectopic pregnancy: risk factors and reproductive outcome: results of a population-based study in France. *Am. J. Obstet. Gynecol.,* 1999; 180: 938.

[35] Dart RG, Kaplan B, Varaklis K. Predictive value of history and physical examination in patients with suspected ectopic pregnancy. *Ann. Emerg. Med.,* 1999; 33:283.

[36] Buckley RG, King KJ, Disney JD, et al. History and physical examination to estimate the risk of ectopic pregnancy: validation of a clinical prediction model. *Ann. Emerg. Med.,* 1999; 34:589.

[37] Tulandi, T. Current protocol for ectopic pregnancy. *Contemp. Obstet. Gynecol.,* 1999; 44:42.

[38] Yao M, Tulandi T. Current status of surgical and nonsurgical management of ectopic pregnancy. *Fertil. Steril.,* 1997; 67:421.

[39] Ankum WM, Van der Veen F, Hamerlynck JV, Lammes FB. Laparoscopy: a dispensable tool in the diagnosis of ectopic pregnancy? *Hum. Reprod.,* 1993; 8:1301.

[40] Gabrielli S, Romero R, Pilu G, et al. Accuracy of transvaginal ultrasound and serum hCG in the diagnosis of ectopic pregnancy. *Ultrasound. Obstet. Gynecol.,* 1992; 2:110.

[41] Kirchler HC, Seebacher S, Alge AA, et al. Early diagnosis of tubal pregnancy: changes in tubal blood flow evaluated by endovaginal color Doppler sonography. *Obstet. Gynecol.,* 1993; 82:561.

[42] Daya S. Human chorionic gonadotropin increase in normal early pregnancy. *Am. J. Obstet. Gynecol.,* 1987; 156:286.

[43] Cole LA. Individual deviations in human chorionic gonadotropin concentrations during pregnancy. *Am. J. Obstet. Gynecol.,* 2011; 204: 349 .e1.

[44] Kadar N, DeCherney AH, Romero R. Receiver operating characteristic (ROC) curve analysis of the relative efficacy of single and serial chorionic gonadotropin determinations in the early diagnosis of ectopic pregnancy. *Fertil. Steril.,* 1982; 37:542.

[45] Barnhart KT, Sammel MD, Rinaudo PF, et al. Symptomatic patients with an early viable intrauterine pregnancy: HCG curves redefined. *Obstet. Gynecol.,* 2004; 104:50.

[46] Silva C, Sammel MD, Zhou L, et al. *Human chorionic gonadotropin profile for women with ectopic pregnancy,* 2006; 107:605.

[47] Kadar N, DeVore G, Romero R. Discriminatory hCG zone: its use in the sonographic evaluation for ectopic pregnancy. *Obstet. Gynecol.,* 1981; 58:156.

[48] Rotmensch S, Cole LA. False diagnosis and needless therapy of presumed malignant disease in women with false-positive human chorionic gonadotropin concentrations. *Lancet,* 2000; 355:712.

[49] Cole LA. Phantom hCG and phantom choriocarcinoma. *Gynecol. Oncol.,* 1998;

[50] Olsen TG, Hubert PR, Nycum LR. Falsely elevated human A1; 98:843.

[51] Paul M, Schaff E, Nichols M. The roles of clinical assessment, human chorionic gonadotropin assays, and ultrasonography in medical abortion practice. *Am. J. Obstet. Gynecol.,* 2000; 183:S34.

[52] Barnhart KT, Simhan H, Kamelle SA. Diagnostic accuracy of ultrasound above and below the beta-hCG discriminatory zone. *Obstet. Gynecol.,* 1999; 94:583.

[53] Condous G, Kirk E, Lu C, et al. Diagnostic accuracy of varying discriminatory zones for the prediction of ectopic pregnancy in women with a pregnancy of unknown location. *Ultrasound Obstet. Gynecol.*, 2005; 26:770.
[54] Seeber BE, Barnhart KT. Suspected ectopic pregnancy. *Obstet. Gynecol.*, 2006; 107:399.
[55] Rausch ME, Barnhart KT. Serum biomarkers for detecting ectopic pregnancy. *Clin. Obstet. Gynecol.*, 2012; 55:418.
[56] Verhaegen J, Gallos ID, van Mello NM, et al. Accuracy of single progesterone test to predict early pregnancy outcome in women with pain or bleeding: meta-analysis of cohort studies. *BMJ*, 2012; 345:e6077.
[57] Perkins SL, Al-Ramahi M, Claman P. Comparison of serum progesterone as an indicator of pregnancy nonviability in spontaneously pregnant emergency room and infertility clinic patient populations. *Fertil. Steril.*, 2000; 73:499.
[58] Lindahl B, Ahlgren M. Identification of chorion villi in abortion specimens. *Obstet. Gynecol.*, 1986; 67:79.
[59] Ries A, Singson P, Bidus M, Barnes JG. Use of the endometrial pipelle in the diagnosis of early abnormal gestations. *Fertil. Steril.*, 2000; 74:593.
[60] Barnhart KT, Gracia CR, Reindl B, Wheeler JE. Usefulness of pipelle endometrial biopsy in the diagnosis of women at risk for ectopic pregnancy. *Am. J. Obstet. Gynecol.*, 2003; 188:906.
[61] Pellerito JS, Taylor KJ, Quedens-Case C, et al. Ectopic pregnancy: evaluation with endovaginal color flow imaging. *Radiology*, 1992; 183:407.
[62] Atri M. Ectopic pregnancy versus corpus luteum cyst revisited: best Doppler predictors. *J. Ultrasound. Med.*, 2003; 22:1181.
[63] Kataoka ML, Togashi K, Kobayashi H, et al. Evaluation of ectopic pregnancy by magnetic resonance imaging. *Hum. Reprod.*, 1999; 14:26 44.
[64] Stovall TG, Kellerman AL, Ling FW, Buster JE. Emergency department diagnosis of ectopic pregnancy. *Ann. Emerg. Med.*, 1990; 19:1098.
[65] Mol BW, van der Veen F, Bossuyt PM. Symptom-free women at increased risk of ectopic pregnancy: should we screen? *Acta. Obstet. Gynecol. Scand.*, 2002; 81:661.
[66] De Los Ríos JF, Castañeda JD, Miryam A. Bilateral ectopic pregnancy. *J. Minim. Invasive. Gynecol.*, 2007; 14:419.

[67] Cepni I, Ocal P, Erkan S, Erzik B. Conservative treatment of cervical ectopic pregnancy with transvaginal ultrasound-guided aspiration and single-dose methotrexate. *Fertil. Steril.,* 2004; 81:1130.

[68] Benson CB, Doubilet PM. Strategies for conservative treatment of cervical ectopic pregnancy. *Ultrasound Obstet. Gynecol.,* 1996; 8:371.

[69] Ushakov FB, Elchalal U, Aceman PJ, Schenker JG. Cervical pregnancy: past and future. *Obstet. Gynecol. Surv.,* 1997; 52:45.

[70] Comstock C, Huston K, Lee W. The ultrasonographic appearance of ovarian ectopic pregnancies. *Obstet. Gynecol.,* 2005; 105:42.

[71] Dilbaz S, Katas B, Demir B, Dilbaz B. Treating cornual pregnancy with a single methotrexate injection: a report of 3 cases. *J. Reprod. Med.,* 2005; 50:141.

[72] Lau S, Tulandi T. Conservative medical and surgical management of interstitial ectopic pregnancy. *Fertil. Steril.,* 1999; 72:207.

[73] Fisch JD, Ortiz BH, Tazuke SI, et al. Medical management of interstitial ectopic pregnancy: a case report and literature review. *Hum. Reprod.,* 1998; 13:1981.

[74] Atrash HK, Friede A, Hogue CJ. Abdominal pregnancy in the United States: frequency and maternal mortality. ObstetGynecol 1987; 69:333.

[75] Dover RW, Powell MC. Management of a primary abdominal pregnancy. *Am. J. Obstet. Gynecol.,* 1995; 172:1603.

[76] Fisch B, Peled Y, Kaplan B, et al. Abdominal pregnancy following in vitro fertilization in a patient with previous bilateral salpingectomy. *Obstet. Gynecol.,* 1996; 88:642.

[77] Onan MA, Turp AB, Saltik A, et al. Primary omental pregnancy: case report. *Hum. Reprod.,* 2005; 20:807.

[78] Varma R, Mascarenhas L, James D. Successful outcome of advanced abdominal pregnancy with exclusive omental insertion. *Ultrasound Obstet. Gynecol.,* 2003; 21:192.

[79] Bernstein HB, Thrall MM, Clark WB. Expectant management of intramural ectopic pregnancy. *Obstet. Gynecol.,* 2001; 97:826.

[80] Shinohara A, Yamada A, Imai A. Rupture of noncommunicating rudimentary uterine horn at 27 weeks' gestation with neonatal and maternal survival. *Int. J. Gynaecol. Obstet.,* 2005; 88:316.

[81] Fernandez H, Lelaidier C, Doumerc S, et al. Nonsurgical treatment of heterotopic pregnancy: a report of six cases. *Fertil. Steril.,* 1993; 60:428.

[82] Goldstein JS, Ratts VS, Philpott T, Dahan MH. Risk of surgery after use of potassium chloride for treatment of tubal heterotopic pregnancy. *Obstet. Gynecol.,* 2006; 107:506.

[83] Doubilet PM, Benson CB, Frates MC, Ginsburg E. Sonographically guided minimally invasive treatment of unusual ectopic pregnancies. *J. Ultrasound. Med.,* 2004; 23:359.

[84] Gyamfi C, Cohen S, Stone JL. Maternal complication of cervical heterotopic pregnancy after successful potassium chloride fetal reduction. *Fertil. Steril.,* 2004; 82:940.

[85] Salomon LJ, Fernandez H, Chauveaud A, et al. Successful management of a heterotopic Caesarean scar pregnancy: potassium chloride injection with preservation of the intrauterine gestation: case report. *Hum. Reprod.,* 2003; 18:189.

[86] Rotas MA, Haberman S, Levgur M. Cesarean scar ectopic pregnancies: etiology, diagnosis, and management. *Obstet. Gynecol.,* 2006; 107:1373.

[87] Vial Y, Petignat P, Hohlfeld P. Pregnancy in a cesarean scar. *Ultrasound Obstet. Gynecol.,* 2000; 16:592.

[88] Ash A, Smith A, Maxwell D. Caesarean scar pregnancy. *BJOG,* 2007; 114:253.

[89] Valley MT, Pierce JG, Daniel TB, Kaunitz AM. Cesarean scar pregnancy: imaging and treatment with conservative surgery. *Obstet. Gynecol.,* 1998; 91:838.

[90] Habbu J, Read MD. Ovarian pregnancy successfully treated with methotrexate. *J. Obstet. Gynaecol.,* 2006; 26:587.

[91] Raziel A, Golan A. Primary ovarian pregnancy successfully treated with methotrexate. *Am. J. Obstet. Gynecol.,* 1993; 169:1362.

[92] Shamma FN, Schwartz LB. Primary ovarian pregnancy successfully treated with methotrexate. *Am. J. Obstet. Gynecol.,* 1992; 167:1307.

[93] Fishman DA, Padilla LA, Joob A, Lurain JR. Ectopic pregnancy causing hemothorax managed by thoracoscopy and actinomycin D. *Obstet. Gynecol.,* 1998; 91:837.

[94] Jansen RP, Elliott PM. Angular intrauterine pregnancy. *Obstet. Gynecol.,* 1981; 58:167.

[95] Larraín D, Marengo F, Bourdel N, et al. Proximal ectopic pregnancy: a descriptive general population-based study and results of different management options in 86 cases. *Fertil. Steril.,* 2011; 95:867.

[96] Tulandi T, Al-Jaroudi D. Interstitial pregnancy: results generated from the Society of Reproductive Surgeons Registry. *Obstet. Gynecol.,* 2004; 103:47.

[97] Soriano D, Vicus D, Mashiach R, et al. Laparoscopic treatment of cornual pregnancy: a series of 20 consecutive cases. *Fertil. Steril., 2008*; 90:839.

[98] LUND J. Early ectopic pregnancy; comments on conservative treatment. *J. Obstet. Gynaecol. Br. Emp.,* 1955; 62:70.

[99] Shalev E, Peleg D, Tsabari A, et al. Spontaneous resolution of ectopic tubal pregnancy: natural history. *Fertil. Steril.,* 1995; 63:15.

[100] Rotas MA, Haberman S, Levgur M. Cesarean scar ectopic pregnancies: etiology, diagnosis, and management. *Obstet. Gynecol.,* 2006; 107:1373.

[101] Vial Y, Petignat P, Hohlfeld P. Pregnancy in a cesarean scar. *Ultrasound Obstet. Gynecol.,* 2000; 16:592.

[102] Ash A, Smith A, Maxwell D. Caesarean scar pregnancy. *BJOG,* 2007; 114:253.

[103] Valley MT, Pierce JG, Daniel TB, Kaunitz AM. Cesarean scar pregnancy: imaging and treatment with conservative surgery. ObstetGynecol 1998; 100.Korhonen J, Stenman UH, Ylöstalo P. Serum human chorionic gonadotropin dynamics during spontaneous resolution of ectopic pregnancy. *Fertil. Steril.,* 1994; 61:632.

[104] Tulandi T, Al-Jaroudi D. Interstitial pregnancy: results generated from the Society of Reproductive Surgeons Registry. *Obstet. Gynecol.,* 2004; 103:47.

[105] Trio D, Strobelt N, Picciolo C, et al. Prognostic factors for successful expectant management of ectopic pregnancy. *Fertil. Steril.,* 1995; 63:469.

[106] Tulandi T, Ferenczy A, Berger E. Tubal occlusion as a result of retained ectopic pregnancy: a case report. *Am. J. Obstet. Gynecol.,* 1988; 158:11 16…

[107] 3 LUND J. Early ectopic pregnancy; comments on conservative treatment. *J. Obstet. Gynaecol. Br. Emp.,* 1955; 62:70.

[108] Yao M, Tulandi T. Current status of surgical and nonsurgical management of ectopic pregnancy. *Fertil. Steril.,* 1997; 67:421.

[109] Kirk E, Condous G, Bourne T. The non-surgical management of ectopic pregnancy. *Ultrasound Obstet. Gynecol.,* 2006; 27:91.

[110] Korhonen J, Stenman UH, Ylostalo P. Low-dose oral methotrexate with expectant management of ectopic pregnancy. *Obstet. Gynecol.,* 1996; 88:775.

[111] American College of Obstetricians and Gynecologists. ACOG Practice Bulletin No. 94: Medical management of ectopic pregnancy. *Obstet. Gynecol.,* 2008; 111:1479.

[112] Trio D, Strobelt N, Picciolo C, et al. Prognostic factors for successful expectant management of ectopic pregnancy. *Fertil. Steril.,* 1995; 63:469.

[113] van Mello NM, Mol F, Verhoeve HR, et al. Methotrexate or expectant management in women with an ectopic pregnancy or pregnancy of unknown location and low serum hCG concentrations? A randomized comparison. *Hum. Reprod.,* 2013; 28:60.

[114] van Mello NM, Mol F, Adriaanse AH, et al. The METEX study: methotrexate versus expectant management in women with ectopic pregnancy: a randomised controlled trial. *BMC Womens Health,* 2008; 8:10.

[115] Banerjee S, Aslam N, Zosmer N, et al. The expectant management of women with early pregnancy of unknown location. *Ultrasound Obstet. Gynecol.,* 1999; 14:231.

[116] 4 Lipscomb GH. Medical therapy for ectopic pregnancy. *Semin. Reprod. Med.,* 2007; 25:93.

[117] Van Den Eeden SK, Shan J, Bruce C, Glasser M. Ectopic pregnancy rate and treatment utilization in a large managed care organization. *Obstet. Gynecol.,* 2005; 105:1052.

[118] Barnhart KT, Gosman G, Ashby R, Sammel M. The medical management of ectopic pregnancy: a meta-analysis comparing "single dose" and "multidose" regimens. *Obstet. Gynecol.,* 2003; 101:778.

[119] Farquhar CM. Ectopic pregnancy. *Lancet,* 2005; 366:583.

[120] Morlock RJ, Lafata JE, Eisenstein D. Cost-effectiveness of single-dose methotrexate compared with laparoscopic treatment of ectopic pregnancy. *Obstet. Gynecol.,* 2000; 95:407.

[121] Bleyer WA. The clinical pharmacology of methotrexate: new applications of an old drug. *Cancer,* 1978; 41:36.

[122] Nilsson UW, Johns TG, Wilmann T, et al. Effects of gefitinib, an epidermal growth factor receptor inhibitor, on human placental cell growth. *Obstet. Gynecol.,* 2013; 122:737.

[123] Skubisz MM, Horne AW, Johns TG, et al. Combination gefitinib and methotrexate compared with methotrexate alone to treat ectopic pregnancy. *Obstet. Gynecol.,* 2013; 122:745.

[124] Practice Committee of the American Society for Reproductive Medicine. Medical treatment of ectopic pregnancy. *Fertil. Steril.,* 2006; 86:S96.

[125] Medical management of ectopic pregnancy. ACOG Practice Bulletin #94.American College of Obstetricians and Gynecologists, 2008.

[126] Kelly H, Harvey D, Moll S. A cautionary tale: fatal outcome of methotrexate therapy given for management of ectopic pregnancy. *Obstet. Gynecol.,* 2006; 107:439.

[127] Teal SB. A cautionary tale: fatal outcome of methotrexate therapy given for management of ectopic pregnancy. ObstetGynecol 2006; 107:1420.
[128] Lipscomb GH, McCord ML, Stovall TG, et al. Predictors of success of methotrexate treatment in women with tubal ectopic pregnancies. *N. Engl. J. Med.*, 1999; 341:1974.
[129] Lipscomb GH, Bran D, McCord ML, et al. Analysis of three hundred fifteen ectopic pregnancies treated with single-dose methotrexate. *Am. J. Obstet. Gynecol.*, 1998; 178:1354.
[130] .Shalev E, Peleg D, Bustan M, et al. Limited role for intratubal methotrexate treatment of ectopic pregnancy. *Fertil. Steril.*, 1995; 63:20.
[131] Nazac A, Gervaise A, Bouyer J, et al. Predictors of success in methotrexate treatment of women with unruptured tubal pregnancies. *Ultrasound Obstet. Gynecol.*, 2003; 21:181.
[132] Doubilet PM, Benson CB, Bourne T, et al. Diagnostic criteria for nonviable pregnancy early in the first trimester. *N. Engl. J. Med.*, 2013; 369:1443.
[133] Stovall TG, Ling FW, Gray LA, et al. Methotrexate treatment of unruptured ectopic pregnancy: a report of 100 cases. *Obstet. Gynecol.*, 1991; 77:749.
[134] .Stovall TG, Ling FW. Single-dose methotrexate: an expanded clinical trial. *Am. J. Obstet. Gynecol.*, 1993; 168:1759.
[135] Stovall TG, Ling FW, Buster JE. Reproductive performance after methotrexate treatment of ectopic pregnancy. *Am. J. Obstet. Gynecol.*, 1990; 162:1620.
[136] Gougeon A. Dynamics of follicular growth in the human: a model from preliminary results. *Hum. Reprod.*, 1986; 1:81.
[137] Strauss, JF, Williams, CJ. The ovarian life cycle. In: Yen and Jaffe's Reproductive Endocrinology: Physiology, Pathophysiology, and Clinical Management, 5th ed, Strauss, JF, Barbieri, RL (Eds), Elsevier Saunders, Philadelphia 2004. p.213.
[138] Pektasides D, Rustin GJ, Newlands ES, et al. Fertility after chemotherapy for ovarian germ cell tumours. *Br. J. Obstet. Gynaecol.*, 1987; 94:477.
[139] Ayhan A, Ergeneli MH, Yuce K, et al. Pregnancy after chemotherapy for gestational trophoblastic disease. *J. Reprod. Med.*, 1990; 35:522.
[140] Keefe KA, Wald JS, Goldstein DP, et al. Reproductive outcome after methotrexate treatment of tubal pregnancies. *J. Reprod. Med.*, 1998; 43:28.

[141] Kung FT, Chang SY, Tsai YC, et al. Subsequent reproduction and obstetric outcome after methotrexate treatment of cervical pregnancy: a review of original literature and international collaborative follow-up. *Hum. Reprod.,* 1997; 12:591.

[142] Oriol B, Barrio A, Pacheco A, et al. Systemic methotrexate to treat ectopic pregnancy does not affect ovarian reserve. *Fertil. Steril.,* 2008; 90:1579.

[143] Wiser A, Gilbert A, Nahum R, et al. Effects of treatment of ectopic pregnancy with methotrexate or salpingectomy in the subsequent IVF cycle. *Reprod. Biomed. Online,* 2013; 26:449.

[144] 5 Yao M, Tulandi T. Current status of surgical and nonsurgical management of ectopic pregnancy. *Fertil. Steril.,* 1997; 67:421.

[145] Hajenius PJ, Mol F, Mol BW, et al. Interventions for tubal ectopic pregnancy. *Cochrane Database Syst. Rev.,* 2007; :CD000324.

[146] Murphy AA, Nager CW, Wujek JJ, et al. Operative laparoscopy versus laparotomy for the management of ectopic pregnancy: a prospective trial. *Fertil. Steril.,* 1992; 57:1180.

[147] Vermesh M, Silva PD, Rosen GF, et al. Management of unruptured ectopic gestation by linear salpingostomy: a prospective, randomized clinical trial of laparoscopy versus laparotomy. *Obstet. Gynecol.,* 1989; 73:400.

[148] Lundorff P, Thorburn J, Hahlin M, et al. Laparoscopic surgery in ectopic pregnancy. A randomized trial versus laparotomy. *Acta. Obstet. Gynecol. Scand.,* 1991; 70:343.

[149] Bangsgaard N, Lund CO, Ottesen B, Nilas L. Improved fertility following conservative surgical treatment of ectopic pregnancy. *BJOG,* 2003; 110:765.

[150] Silva PD, Schaper AM, Rooney B. Reproductive outcome after 143 laparoscopic procedures for ectopic pregnancy. *Obstet. Gynecol.,* 1993; 81:710.

[151] Job-Spira N, Bouyer J, Pouly JL, et al. Fertility after ectopic pregnancy: first results of a population-based cohort study in france. *Hum. Reprod.,* 1996; 11:99.

[152] Mol BW, Matthijsse HC, Tinga DJ, et al. Fertility after conservative and radical surgery for tubal pregnancy. *Hum. Reprod.,* 1998; 13:1804.

[153] Dubuisson JB, Morice P, Chapron C, et al. Salpingectomy - the laparoscopic surgical choice for ectopic pregnancy. *Hum. Reprod.,* 1996; 11:1199.

[154] Savaris RF, Cavazzola LT. Ectopic pregnancy: laparoendoscopic single-site surgery--laparoscopic surgery through a single cutaneous incision. *Fertil. Steril.*, 2009; 92:1170.e5.

[155] Lee ES, Hahn HS, Park BJ, et al. Single-port laparoscopic cornual resection for a spontaneous cornual ectopic pregnancy following ipsilateral salpingectomy. *Fertil. Steril.*, 2011; 96:e106.

[156] Lazard A, Poizac S, Courbiere B, et al. Cornual resection for interstitial pregnancy by laparoendoscopic single-site surgery. *Fertil. Steril.*, 2011; 95:2432.e5.

[157] Bedaiwy MA, Escobar PF, Pinkerton J, Hurd W. Laparoendoscopic single-site salpingectomy in isthmic and ampullary ectopic pregnancy: preliminary report and technique. *J. Minim. Invasive. Gynecol.*, 2011; 18:230.

[158] Yoon BS, Park H, Seong SJ, et al. Single-port versus conventional laparoscopic salpingectomy in tubal pregnancy: a comparison of surgical outcomes. *Eur. J. Obstet. Gynecol. Reprod. Biol.*, 2011; 159:190.

[159] Tulandi T. Tubal ectopic pregnancy: salpingostomy and salpingectomy. In: Atlas of Laparoscopy and Hysteroscopy Technique, Tulandi T (Ed), WB Saunders Co, London 1999. p.49.

[160] Tulandi T, Guralnick M. Treatment of tubal ectopic pregnancy by salpingotomy with or without tubal suturing and salpingectomy. *Fertil. Steril.*, 1991; 55:53.

[161] Fujishita A, Masuzaki H, Khan KN, et al. Laparoscopic salpingotomy for tubal pregnancy: comparison of linear salpingotomy with and without suturing. *Hum. Reprod.*, 2004; 19:1195.

[162] Lau S, Tulandi T. Conservative medical and surgical management of interstitial ectopic pregnancy. *Fertil. Steril.*, 1999; 72:207.

[163] Habana A, Dokras A, Giraldo JL, Jones EE. Cornual heterotopic pregnancy: contemporary management options. *Am. J. Obstet. Gynecol.*, 2000; 182:1264.

[164] Moon HS, Choi YJ, Park YH, Kim SG. New simple endoscopic operations for interstitial pregnancies. *Am. J. Obstet. Gynecol.*, 2000; 182:114.

[165] Moawad NS, Mahajan ST, Moniz MH, et al. Current diagnosis and treatment of interstitial pregnancy. *Am. J. Obstet. Gynecol.*, 2010; 202:15.

[166] Tulandi T, Al-Jaroudi D. Interstitial pregnancy: results generated from the Society of Reproductive Surgeons Registry. *Obstet. Gynecol.*, 2004; 103:47.

[167] Stovall TG, Ling FW, Buster JE. Outpatient chemotherapy of unruptured ectopic pregnancy. *Fertil. Steril.,* 1989; 51:435.
[168] Jermy K, Thomas J, Doo A, Bourne T. The conservative management of interstitial pregnancy. *BJOG,* 2004; 111:1283.
[169] Soriano D, Vicus D, Mashiach R, et al. Laparoscopic treatment of cornual pregnancy: a series of 20 consecutive cases. *Fertil. Steril.,* 2008; 90:839.
[170] Meyer WR, Mitchell DE. Hysteroscopic removal of an interstitial ectopic gestation.A case report. *J. Reprod. Med.,* 1989; 34:928.
[171] Budnick SG, Jacobs SL, Nulsen JC, Metzger DA. Conservative management of interstitial pregnancy. *Obstet. Gynecol. Surv.,* 1993; 48:694.
[172] Weissman A, Fishman A. Uterine rupture following conservative surgery for interstitial pregnancy. *Eur. J. Obstet. Gynecol. Reprod. Biol.,* 1992; 44:237.
[173] Downey GP, Tuck SM. Spontaneous uterine rupture during subsequent pregnancy following non-excision of an interstitial ectopic gestation. Br *J. Obstet. Gynaecol.,* 1994; 101:162.
[174] Farquhar CM. Ectopic pregnancy. *Lancet,* 2005; 366:583.
[175] .Spandorfer SD, Sawin SW, Benjamin I, Barnhart KT. Postoperative day 1 serum human chorionic gonadotropin level as a predictor of persistent ectopic pregnancy after conservative surgical management. *Fertil. Steril.,* 1997; 68:430.
[176] .Gracia CR, Brown HA, Barnhart KT. Prophylactic methotrexate after linear salpingostomy: a decision analysis. *Fertil. Steril.,* 2001; 76:1191.
[177] Seifer DB, Silva PD, Grainger DA, et al. Reproductive potential after treatment for persistent ectopic pregnancy. *Fertil. Steril.,* 1994; 62:194.
[178] Ego A, Subtil D, Cosson M, et al. Survival analysis of fertility after ectopic pregnancy. *Fertil. Steril.,* 2001; 75:560.
[179] Gervaise A, Masson L, de Tayrac R, et al. Reproductive outcome after methotrexate treatment of tubal pregnancies. *Fertil. Steril.,* 2004; 82:304.
[180] Tulandi T. Reproductive performance of women after two tubal ectopic pregnancies. *Fertil. Steril.,* 1988; 50:164.
[181] .Ory SJ, Nnadi E, Herrmann R, et al. Fertility after ectopic pregnancy. *Fertil. Steril.,* 1993; 60:231.
[182] Sultana CJ, Easley K, Collins RL. Outcome of laparoscopic versus traditional surgery for ectopic pregnancies. *Fertil. Steril.,* 1992; 57:285.

[183] .Pouly JL, Chapron C, Manhes H, et al. Multifactorial analysis of fertility after conservative laparoscopic treatment of ectopic pregnancy in a series of 223 patients. *Fertil.Steril.,* 1991; 56:453.
[184] Bernoux A, Job-Spira N, Germain E, et al. Fertility outcome after ectopic pregnancy and use of an intrauterine device at the time of the index ectopic pregnancy. *Hum. Reprod.,* 2000; 15:1173.
[185] Dubuisson JB, Aubriot FX, Foulot H, et al. Reproductive outcome after laparoscopic salpingectomy for tubal pregnancy. *Fertil. Steril.,* 1990; 53:1004.

In: Ectopic Pregnancy
Editor: Mallory T. Church

ISBN: 978-1-63463-260-7

Chapter 6

A Review of Rare Reproductive Dysfunctions: A Complex Phenomenon of Mammals and Women

Eduardo Tena-Betancourt[1,2,*], *Braulio Hernández-Godínez*[3], *Alejandra Ibáñez-Contreras*[3], *Verónica Graullera-Rivera*[4] *and Daniel Muñoz-Jiménez*[1]

[1]Animal Facility Services and Experimental Surgery, Mexican Faculty of Medicine, La Salle University, Mexico
[2]Department of Ethology, Wildlife and Laboratory Animals, Faculty of Veterinary Medicine and Zootechnics, Mexico
[3]BIOINVERT®. Biología Integral para Vertebrados: Unidad de Experimentación Animal, Mexico
[4] Department of Pathology, INC "Ignacio Chávez", Mexico

[*] Corresponding author: E-mail: eduardo.tena@ulsa.mx.

Abstract

In human reproduction term pregnancy is the normal, expected outcome that culminates with the delivery of healthy descendants. The distinctive phenomenon of reproduction occurs amid a complex array of molecular, genetic, metabolic and hormonal influences contributing to successful pregnancies, although this process does not always evolves normally and highly disturbed outcomes have been reported as medical rarities since ancient times. In modern medicine, frequent accounts of rare reproductive disorders such as pregnancy loss due to Ectopic Pregnancy (EP), constitute one of the most devastating medical concerns of the last 35 years, having not only a negative impact by compromising fertility among young women but resulting also in considerable fatalities signifying great economic burden on societies world-wide. Given the alarming demographic increases of reproductive dysfunctions major ethically acceptable research efforts have been devised in humans and animal models, as they comprise an important medical tool where ongoing research has proven to be of great value to define a better understanding of complex genetic, immunologic, hormonal and metabolic factors leading to EP in women, when unknown disturbances deregulate embryotubal transport and tubal microenvironment is modified, suggesting the need to further study multifaceted risk factors of fetal loss in alternative animal models such as lagomorphs and swine, species where major discoveries have been documented. Finally, the objective of this chapter is to contribute to the current knowledge of reproductive anomalies disclosing novel related risk factors described in research in animal models, and discuss an analogous panorama of EP in the rabbit, a species that has provided well-documented rarities encompassing fetal complications and constitute a unique potential source of research resources.

Keywords: Pregnancy loss, Tubal Implantation, Research, Abdominal Pregnancy, Lithopedia, Morphological Characterization

Introduction

Human reproduction is one of the most important wonders of God's creation as it was biblically documented in Genesis, Chapter I (Ohlman 2010). Such a precious gift stands for the sole principle of life as we know it and has been the subject of countless mystical narratives in art since the early history of medicine (Petralia and Bertini 2010).

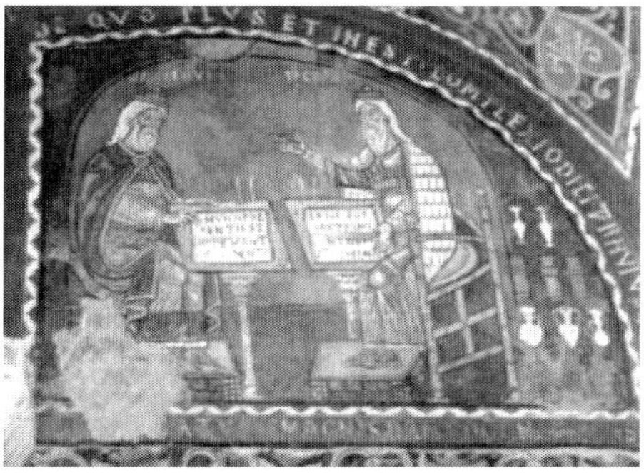

Photo: Nina Aldin Thune. Reprinted with permission.

Figure 1. Hippocrates and Galen.

The classical writings of ancient Egyptians (David 2004) discussed the womb as a source of diverse bodily symptoms; analysis of translations of the Ebers, Berlin, Carlsberg and Kahun Gynaecological Papyri revealed profound knowledge of reproductive issues and contraception among Egyptian midwifes, including extraordinary series of fertility tests and to determine the sex of the unborn child (Hasan 2011). Several exceptional medical advances usually attributed to the Greeks by modern research can be traced back in earlier Egyptian medical traditions, which described *'rational' and 'irrational'* procedures (David 2008). The disturbances of the uterus, a unique privileged place for new life, have been extensively narrated by great medical philosophers such as Hippocrates (Merskey et al., 1993), who in a collection of writings (460 to 370 BC) included detailed sections dealing with hysteria, considered the root of women's mental health (Figure 1).

By conceiving the term "hysteria" (from the Greek word for uterus, *hystera*), Hippocrates explained specific mental conditions originating from perturbation of the uterus (Lim et al., 2010). In today's medicine it has long been known that the uterus does not contribute to such psychological problems, but it rather remains a complex source of distinct female-specific pathologic, life-threatening health conditions in women and animals.

As the only means for perpetuation in the species, reproduction has always been a fascinating theme occurring amidst a broad spectrum of obscure phenomena, for the most part described as obstetric rarities since the times of ancient Egyptians and Greeks (Rabinerson et al., 2008), who reported naturally-occurring spontaneous events, or after a misconception occurred in human or animal reproduction (Kobayashi et al., 1996).

Anatomically, the uterus forms part of the urogenital system but early development rests on fundamental embryonic processes leading to the formation of oviducts, uterus, cervix, and the upper portion of the vagina amid complex genetic processes that influence its development and life-time functionality (Kobayashi et al., 2003). The additive or multiplicative role of modifier genes greatly influences the presence of metabolic diseases and human malformations, as it has been reported in human development and animal malformation syndromes in addition to multifactorial diseases (Slavotinek et al., 2003; Saifudeen et al., 2012). The distinctive reproductive function of the uterus is strictly regulated by regular cycles of ovarian sex steroid hormones influencing cyclic endometrial cell changes; any genetically-determined or hormonal alteration can adversely compromise fertility, since once oocyte fertilization takes place the reproductive tract supports further development of the fetus, and provides the passage for birth (Kobayashi et al., 2003).

Since profound ethical concerns have imposed a restriction to the study of human pregnancy and developmental changes, most research dealt with basic biology and clinical case-reports; therefore, researchers have resorted to use animal models to study mammalian reproductive biology functions and infrequent rarities such as malformations.

The aim of this work is to further contribute to the current knowledge of reproductive anomalies by highlighting novel-related risk factors described in animal models, and to discuss a comparable panorama of EP in the rabbit, species where analogous, pregnancy rarities and complications have been observed.

Pregnancy Complications

Term pregnancy is the usual, expected scenario among pregnant mammals. Nevertheless, it has been reported that any hormonal, genetic or embryonic demise might lead to dysfunction of pregnancy amid a complex unbalance of various delicate phases resulting in pregnancy loss, possibly associated to various factors such as chromosomal aberration, poor implantation, early undernourishment or metabolic and immunological diseases or resulting in ectopic pregnancy (EP) among other dysfunctions (Lim et al., 2010). The multifaceted risk factors of fetal loss due to EP remain inconclusive and reports suggest that apparently no suitable animal model has been reported, restricting the study of this rarity to human medicine when is ethically appropriate (Lim et al., 2010). Nevertheless, experimental debatable approaches have studied the effect of toxic carcinogens such as DAB-4HCL (3-3'-Diaminobenzidine tetrahydrochloride[1]) on pregnant does, inducing severe policythemia, leukocytosis, enzymatic and hormonal changes to induce EP (Aliawy 2010).

Alternative research has demonstrated the role of inhibitory factors which play a critical role suppressing embryo viability and tubal implantation in rabbits, by eliciting an embryo-dormancy-inducing factor in obstructed healthy mouse oviducts impeding EP (Lee et al., 2000; Lin et al., 2001).

In this section we would elaborate about experimental EP and its spontaneous occurrence in animal models, basically the rabbit, considered a unique model employed among other alternative species in assisted reproduction since the work of L. Spallanzani (1784), who achieved the first successful artificial insemination (AI) in a dog (Foote 2002). Other significant use of this species is credited to Walter Heape, a professor at the University of Cambridge, UK, who reported the first known case of embryo transplantation in rabbits as early as 1890 (Kamel et al., 2013). Such data and further work lead to the creation of a world center for reproductive studies in Cambridge UK (Foote 2002).

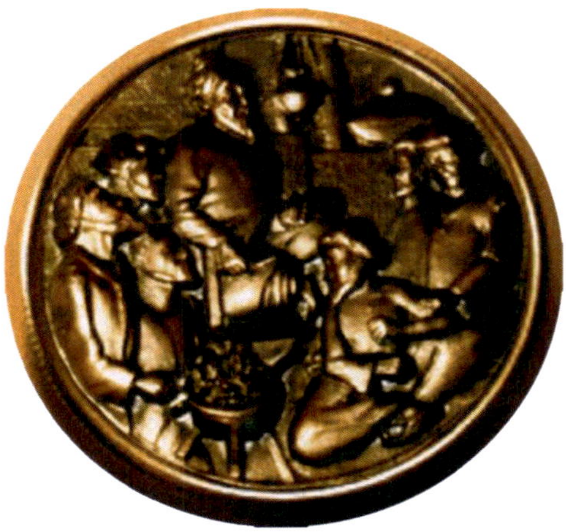

Figure 2. Commemorating Medal – The Millennium Anniversary, Al-Zahrawi (Albucasis)[2].

[1] DAB-4HCL - Material Safety Data Sheet. Polysciences, Inc., 400 Valley Road Warrington, PA 18976. Phone. (215) 343-6484.

The Rarity of Ectopic Pregnancy

Ectopic pregnancy (EP) is an unexpected, relatively uncommon occurrence in most mammalian species and women (Rana et al., 2013; Corpa 2006). Ancient writings indicate that this pathology was recognized well over 900 years ago by Albucassis (930-1013 AD), an Andalusian medic considered the greatest medieval surgeon of the Islamic World, (Ahmad 2007) and the first physician to describe EP among other discoveries of hereditary nature (Cosman, et al., 2008). Given its early transcendental work in medicine the world community of scholars celebrated a millennium after his death in 1013, and recognized him as the renowned Andalusian physician-surgeon Abu al-Qasim al-Zahrawi (Abulcasis) in 2013. An editorial was Posted on January 20, 2014[2].

The term ectopic derives from the Greek word *´Ektopos´*, meaning out of place indicating implantation of a fertilized egg outside the uterine cavity as reported by Bland-Sutton (1994). Being an obstetric rarity EP was quoted by Buckley and Caine (1979) as the leading cause of high maternal morbidity, fetal loss and substantial medical and economic consequences that resulted in alarming epidemiologic reports (Coste et al., 2004; Nour, FOM 2010).

World-wide incidence rates of EP vary enormously depending upon geographical sites (Coste et al., 2000; Coste et al., 2004). Several epidemiological trends place EP as a serious pathology linked to pelvic inflammatory disease (PID) and tubal factor infertility, and the leading cause of maternal mortality and catastrophic medical care costs (Rana et al., 2013; Creanga et al., 2011; Tay, et al., 2000; Simms et al., 1997). When EP is misdiagnosed delaying early treatment, severe morbidity or mortality results and future fertility may be compromised among young adult women (Shafi, et al., 2009; Van Den et al., 2005; Atrash et al., 1987).

Reports indicate that EP has evolved over recent decades showing serious increases in European countries (Rajkhowa et al., 2000; Tay, et al., 2000). A dramatic increase of EP cases has been recorded in US hospitals since 1970; during a period of 19 years the number of admissions related to EP increased more than 400% to 18,000 (Simms et al., 1997; CDC (1995); CDC (1992); CDC (1988). Being a serious miscarriage threat, guidelines aimed to aid in the diagnosis and early management of pregnancy to avoid unnecessary deaths have been published elsewhere (Newbatt et al., 2012).

---

[2] Adapted from: http://www.muslimheritage.com/article/millennium-anniversary-abu-al-qasim-al- zahrawi.

In order to describe EP a few criteria have been considered to define its morphologic features and enable accurate diagnosis (Corpa 2006). If classified by its type of presentation (Figure 3), four types are distinguished: tubaric, ovaric, abdominal or peritoneal and cervical, being the fallopian tube the commonest location (97%), known as tubal pregnancy (TB), where implantation can occur at any point along the tube although the ampullar is the most frequent site (Complications of Pregnancy Part 1, 2007; Coste et al., 2005). Depending on the location where implantation takes place, subtypes of fimbrial (17%), ampullar (55%) and isthmic (25%) EP has been acknowledged. A further classification defines gestation developing in the peritoneal cavity as abdominal pregnancy (AP) as is divided into primary and secondary (Tena et al., 2013; Corpa 2006; Segura-Gil, et al., 2004).

Primary AP defines that fertilization must have occurred outside the uterus, where an oocyte is accidentally released from the fimbrial or the oviduct segments, is fertilized and develops primitively attached to a proper placental structure and viscera leading to the formation of lithopedions (from the Greek (*λίθος* = stone; *παιδός* = child); secondary AP is the direct result of tubaric trauma and mostly occurs undetected allowing implantation to take place randomly within the abdomen, viscera or ligaments (Segura-Gil et al., 2004; Tay et al., 2000). One extremely rare form of EP is heterotopic, when two fertilized eggs co-exist, one outside the uterus and the other inside; this rarity is associated with high maternal morbidity and fetal mortality and to date no animal reports are available (Adesiyun et al., 2012; Aliyu et al., 2008; Odewale, et al., 2008).

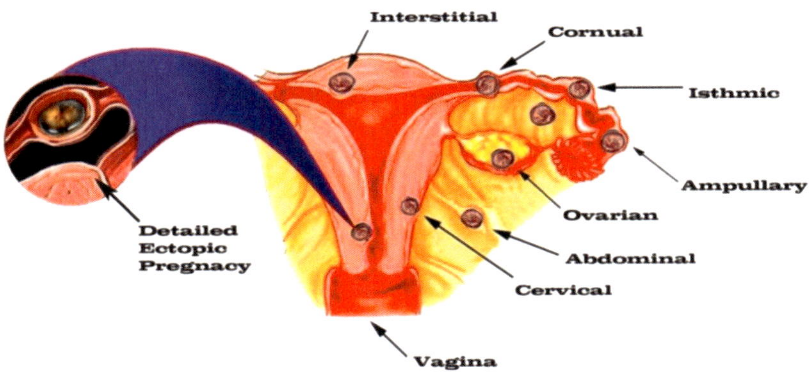

Figure adapted from: http://primitive-streak.org/images/implantation3.jpg, http:// allaboutreproductivehealth.wordpress.com/

Figure 3. Common Sites of Human Ectopic Pregnancy.

In laboratory animals remarkable examples of EP have been documented (Eales 1932); one of the first papers written as early as 1904 by Bland-Sutton (1904) reporting comparative abdominal pregnancies in women, cats, dogs and rabbits among the most frequently affected (Segura-Gil et al., 2004); although a high incidence of multiple AP was described by Buckley and Caine A. (1979) in Dunjarian hamsters (*Phodopus sungorus*).

Additional reports revealed that EP has been occasionally encountered in dogs (Eddey 2012) and other domestic animals, where a case of full-term viable lambs was recorded (Mitchell 1989).

Among small rodents tubaric or ovaric EP has been reported in rats (Gosden 1981) and a low incidence in cavies (Hong 1978), with accounts of completely developed ectopic fetuses (Araujo 1964). Although relatively rare in feline practice, EP have occurred classified as spontaneous or secondary associated to post-surgical neutering, trauma or genital infections (Rosset et al., 2011; Hannon CA 1981; McKeating 1979; Crownover and Yeargan 1976; McClure and Chang 1975). In nonhuman primates, only a few cases of tubal pregnancies have been recorded among 3000 pregnancies of monkeys described by Lapin, et al., (1963) but it has been occasionally reported in some primate species (Krugner-Higby et al., 2009; Schlabritz-Loutsevitch, et al., 2004; Bunte and Hildebrandt 1975). Despite the number of animal species in which EP implantation has been observed it is remarkable that EP had not elicited obvious clinical signs, nor interfered with reproduction during its late stages leading to the formation of lithopedions.

Experimental Ectopic Implantation in Animal Models

According to Carlton et al., (1991), there is a virtual absence of spontaneous tubal pregnancy in animals that seem to have an effective ability to avoid tubal pregnancy. Several attempts have been reported in the experimental field, but animal models in which tubal ectopic pregnancy can be replicated have proved difficult to develop.

In the experimental field, mouse embryos were successfully transferred to a variety of sites in rodents (Figure 4) including the peritoneal cavity, kidney, spleen, muscles, testis and the anterior chamber of the eye, experimented also in the rabbit (Bland and Donovan 1965; Hreshchyshyn and Hreshchyshyn (1964); Ahlgren and Bengtsson (1962); Fawcett et al., 1947).

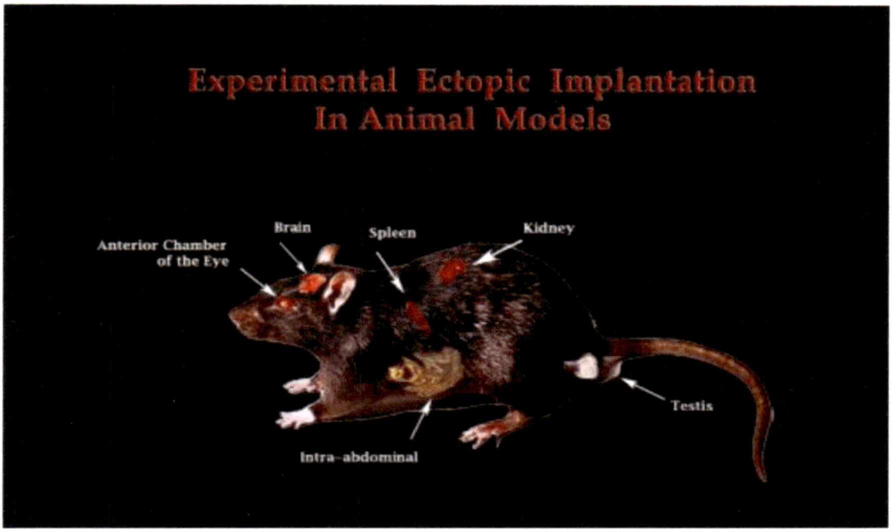

Adapted by Example: Fawcett et al. 1947, Ahlgren et al. 1962, Bland, et al. 1965.

Figure 4. Graphic Representation of Experimental Ectopic Implantation in a Murine Model.

Rationale of EP and Reproductive Dysfunctions in Small Mammals

The common practice of breeding rabbits has been perpetuated in most countries, where inbred, random bred and other breeding patterns are employed by veterinarians and farmers to produce rabbits as laboratory animals and meat, due to its known nutritional health properties and the possible oxidative stability of rabbit meat (Dalle Zotte and Szendrö 2011; Choi et al., 2004). When reproductive disorders are observed, they frequently consist of silent occurrences where different scenarios have been clinically illustrated in rabbits (Tena-Betancourt et al., 2014; Corpa 2006; Harcourt-Brown 2002; Harper et al., 1982).

Early symptoms are rarely observed and vary from sudden death by dystocia, or include unexpected outcomes such as neonatal death of the offspring due to agalactia demanding further clinical assessments (Flecknell 2000). The early stages of pregnancy loss in rabbits seem to occur without previous symptoms analogous to women cases (Tena-Betancourt et al., 2014; Levasseur 1983).

Breeding does might display good health and remain alert and afebrile, and pregnancy loss is often associated to a history of neglected offspring by unknown causes (Bishop 2002; Flecknell 2000; Flatt R.E., Weisbroth S.H., Kraus A.L., 1974). Further physical examination of reported EP cases have revealed pronounced bilateral abdominal distension and the detection of several firm masses of roughly equal size scattered in the abdominal cavity (Tena-Betancourt et al., 2014; Eshar and Mayer 2008). Neither vaginal discharge nor pain is usually reported during palpation, and if fetal death is suspected confirmatory radiographs are usually taken (Dickie 2011).

Radiographic confirmation of ectopic masses has been reported in comprehensive studies as highly mobile, attached or non-attached to internal organs and invariably leading to the formation of lithopedia (Tena et al., 1991).

Further reports have described (Figure 5) discernible abdominal projections of several interposed skeletal structures of near-term developed fetuses, with detailed vertebrae, ribs, radius, ulna and other bones ex-utero, or compact masses shown with extraordinary detail (Tena-Betancourt et al., 2014).

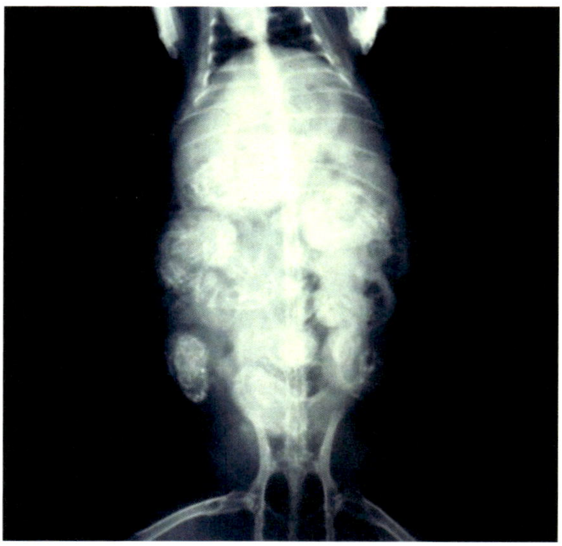

Reprinted with permission.

Figure 5. V.D. Radiograph of a NZW rabbit doe. Mummified fetuses and bony structures are observed ex-utero.

Morphologic Findings in EP

The hallmark of clinical and pathological findings of EP is fetal mummification (Tena-Betancourt et al., 2014). Findings usually revealed one or several mummified fetuses within the uteri or in the abdominal cavity, which vary in size and are observed as solid-scattered bodies floating or attached over the mesentery (Corpa 2006; Eshar and Mayer 2008; Arvidsson 1998).

In rabbits, the number of lithopedions has been reported to be as high as 10 fetuses of more in one or two consecutive pregnancies sharing the same maternal environment (Tena et al., 1991).

A recent report described remarkable, differentiated development of lithopedions ranging from 2.5 to 9.4 cm in total corporal lengths (crown-rump); such findings were analogously compared with valid human scores in order to define to a certain extent preterm growth rates, unavailable for small animal practice (Sasidharan et al., 2009) (Figure 6).

In such approach, size disparity was attributed to age difference among fetuses showing different degrees of maceration, and suggesting that they belong to separate pregnancies (Tena-Betancourt et al., 2014; Eshar and Mayer 2008).

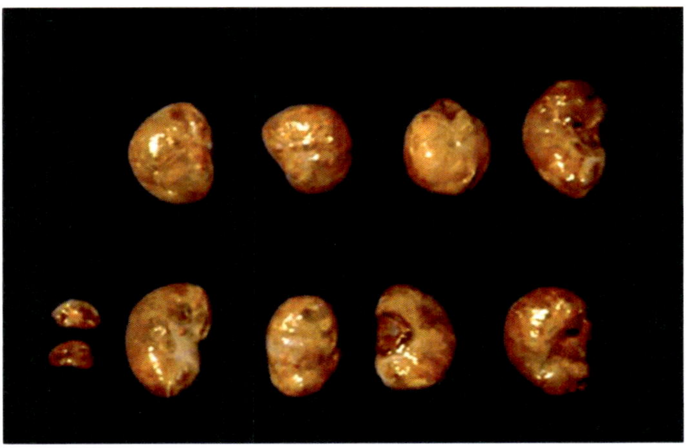

Reprinted with permission.

Figure 6. Lithopedions in a NZW rabbit doe. Note mummification discrepancy; no amniotic fluid is present in the encapsulated chorioallantoic sacs.

Frequently, fetal morphology usually fails to demonstrated true adhesions to nearby mesentery and other abdominal organs; instead, discreet or distinctive attachments have been described as minute thread-like blood vessels linking lithopedions to internal abdominal surfaces (Tena-Betancourt et al., 2014; Segura-Gil 2004; Arvidsson 1998). Nevertheless, an alternative scenario was reported by Harper and Ensley (1982) who described placental remnants firmly adhered to specific segments of the uterus.

Membrane integrity is a common finding in lithopedia; removal of the closely adhered remains of allantois have allowed observing growth differentiation among near-term fetuses which lie down in fetal position and appear curled up inside, having small remnants of a short primitive umbilical cord, individual toes, some hair and whiskers in their faces with both eyes closed (Tena-Betancourt et al., 2014; Corpa 2006) (Figure 7).

In most cases of EP in rabbits, it has been determined that if considered primary, gross examination of the uteri can exhibit normal morphology of outer vascular structures and both ovaries, with no anatomic changes or hematomas. Other morphologic features such as redness, tactile consistency and size have been regarded as normal without evidence of scar formation or recent rupture, grossly and microscopically, which in secondary EP would be present (Tena-Betancourt et al., 2014).

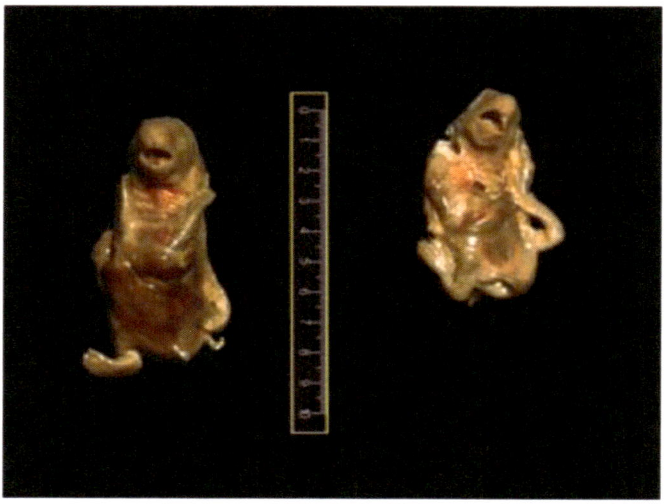

Reprinted with permission.

Figure 7. Dissected lithopedions. Note near-term development, advanced maceration and remnants of primitive umbilical cord and individual toes.

Discussion

Reproduction, the natural intriguing process employed by humans and mammals for their perpetuation is a fascinating theme that occurs amidst a broad spectrum of obscure phenomena (Aliyu et al., 2008; Rabinerson et al., 2008; Pisarska 1998) described as naturally-occurring obstetric rarities since the times of the ancient Greeks (Ohlman 2010; Petralia and Bertini 2010). In women, EP represents a 'life threatening' condition leading to maternal death during early pregnancy (Rana et al., 2013; Odewale and Afolabi 2008; Van Den et al., 2005). While risk factors have been somehow identified, complex molecular mechanisms involved remain to be clarified (Rana et al., 2013; Newbatt, 2010; Nour, 2010).

Genital infections have been accounted as important factors of EP being associated to tubal infertility, as bacteria have been confirmed as a source of oviductal scars (Shao 2010). Lifestyle has been associated as a great concern among users of habitual marijuana, since it has been reported as capable of increasing the risk of ectopic pregnancies by dysregulating endocannabinoid signaling, which disturbs the delicate balance of oviductal smooth muscle contraction and relaxation critical to normal oviductal embryo transport in mice (Lim and Wang 2010; Wang et al., 2004).

While EP symptoms can be considered serious in most human cases, still other underlying causes of embryo retention in the fallopian tube or other ectopic locations remain unidentified. Reports of EP in animal models consistently fail to show early or advanced symptoms of EP, although the basic mechanisms of pregnancy seems to play a critical role given that in mammals the functional integrity of the fallopian tube is estrogen-dependent, possibly influencing tubal functions and embryo transport to the uterus (Kaygusuz et al., 2014; Shao, 2010).

Such assertion leaves no doubt that further animal research might uncover an array of exploration possibilities to enhance current knowledge of the regulatory mechanisms of the vascular endothelial growth factor, placental growth factor expression, secretion, and the role of signaling pathways involved in the pathophysiology of EP among other factors (Shaw et al., 2013; Tay et al., 2000).

In rabbits, data on disorders associated with reproduction are scarce and frequently neglected or ignored by common breeders. It has been observed that well-characterized cases of pseudopregnancy, abortion, pregnancy toxemia and superfetation (SF) displaying remarkable differences in terms of corporal total length and the development of newborn rabbits (Figure 8) have been documented (Tena-Betancourt 2012; Tena-Betancourt 2013). Other reproductive discoveries have included episodes of agalactia (Bishop 2002; Flecknell 2000), congenital or developmental defects (Arendar and Milch 1996) and rarities as ectopic pregnancies (Tena 1991) (Flatt R.E., Weisbroth S.H., Kraus A.L., 1974). Such condition is considered a rarity in any non-marsupial species while its medical significance has been extensively reported in humans and animals (Corpa 2006; Segura-Gil 2004).

Cases of undetected EP leading to the remarkable phenomenon of lithopedia occur when a silent pregnancy takes place intra-abdominally, after fertilized retrograde oocytes are released through the fimbriated portion of the fallopian tube, events occurring in a preceding unknown space of time resulting in EP, which facilitates the differentiated development of lithopedions usually under a silent process analogous to human cases (Tena-Betancourt 2014; Corpa 2006).

Multiple primary EP demonstrating the notorious morphologic development of lithopedions have been confirmed by radiography showing discernible bony fetal structures consistent with near-term fetuses (Tena-Betancourt 2014). Data have included concurrent, smaller soft-fibrous encapsulated fetuses sharing the same sterile abdominal environment, which protects the mother from infection (Tena-Betancourt 2014; Eshar and Mayer 2008). Placental insufficiency seems to be a common finding followed by death and mummification of lithopedions having discernible size disparity, suggesting separate pregnancies (Tena-Betancourt 2014; Owensby et al., 2001; Eshar and Mayer 2008).

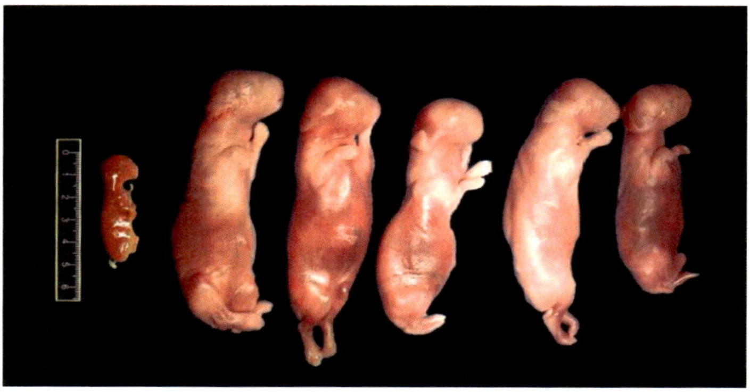

Figure 8. Superfetation in a NZW rabbit doe. Note one single underdeveloped newborn kit (total crown-rump length CRL) among a normal offspring discovered during a cesarean section.

Data shows that since no current animal records are available to compare developmental growth of lithopedions, analogous comparison have been used (Sasidharan et al., 2009) and compared with human scores (Tena-Betancourt, 2014). Early rare accounts of EP have been documented by Eales (1932) and Kuntz (1922) but scarce clinical information was noted.

The characterization of EP in animals might or not be a silent event; usually, intensive reproduction is commonplace in rabbit colonies where symptoms are scarce or so mild that do not trigger serious health conditions, and therefore no interest is attracted among breeders and professional farmers, whose immediate goal is meat production.

According to Segura-Gil P. et al. (2004), intensive Artificial Insemination (AI) protocols could be a factor to consider in EP, as AP incidence was higher in rabbit farms where such practices are common in Spain.

Other additive effects of EP may include the prevalent continuous multiparous character of older does under intensive breeding, accounting as an analogous fact to age and parity observed in women (Pulkkinen 1995).

The clinical features of EP vary among rabbits (Eshar and Mayer 2008; Flecknell 2000; Flatt R.E., Weisbroth S.H., Kraus A.L., 1974). When mild symptoms are acknowledged in breeding does a typical occurrence is sudden death of the nurslings, concomitant to gradual or sudden decay of milk yield impeding optimal sustain of nutritional demands of the suckling kits (Maertens, et al. 2006). If obvious signs exist, these may include severe distress due to fetal load, probably resulting from an unknown form of stress induced by the presence of numerous lithopedions in the dam (Tena-Betancourt, 2014). The temporary lack of appetite and lethargy are notorious in the dams; when palpated, freely moveable or firmly attached masses are felt adhered to some abdominal structures, but palpation does not elicit any signs of pain or discomfort. Also, even if an ongoing silent EP occurs, it has been observed that adequate vulvar conditions can be present and dams readily accept mating followed by excellent nesting behavior suggesting the need of further research.

Conclusion

In human and animal reproduction, factors associated with EP have been a long standing research theme. Current evidence had defined risk factors in woman and animal models with limited experimental responses, suggesting the need to further study this condition and design a clearer didactical approach to better describe this obstetric pathology. Ethical concerns have imposed restrictions on the study of human pregnancy and developmental changes, making it possible that research in murine, lagomorphs and swine models might uncover in the foreseeable future how potential hormonal, genetic and molecular risk factors may be considered by extrapolation of animal research findings to human subjects, affected by certain lifestyles, thus providing a deeper insight to the possible causes of EP, although other related stressors remain to be clarified in breeding dams by way of major efforts in AI research. With that in mind, a wide-scope endeavor should address indigenous infections, malnutrition, fetal load, age and parity, as potential risk factors that appear to be critical and might constitute study targets aimed to enhance the knowledge of the primary pathophysiology of EP. Available breeding resources might promote a large-scale opportunity for future research and cooperation among breeders, mostly unaware of the impact that this interesting field holds in their hands for the advance of medicine.

References

Adesiyun, A. and Ayodele-Cole, B. 2012. Heterotopic tubal pregnancy with live twin birth complicating ovulation induction assisted cycle. *Open J. of Obs. and Gynecol.* 2:325-27. doi: 10.4236/ojog.2012.23068.

Ahlgren, M., Bengtsson, L. P. 1962. Transplantation of fertilized rabbit eggs to the anterior chamber of the eye. *J. Reprod. Fertil.* 3:89-92.

Ahmad, Z. 2007. "Al-Zahrawi - The Father of Surgery", *ANZ J. of Surg.* 77 (Suppl. 1): A83.

Aliawy, A. 2010. Sh. Study to induce ectopic pregnancy by diaminobenzine in Rabbits. *AL-Qadisiya J. Vet. Med. Sci.* 9(2): 37-44.

Aliyu, J. A., Eigbefoh, J. O., Mabayoje, P. S. 2008. Heterotropic Pregnancy: A Report of Two Cases. *Nigerian J. of Clin. Pract.* 11(1): 85-87.

Araujo, P. A case of ectopic abdominal pregnancy in guinea pig. 1964. *Lab. Anim. Care* 14:1-5.

Arendar, G. M., Milch, R. A. 1966. Splay-leg–a recessively inherited form of femoral neck anteversion, femoral shaft torsion, and subluxation of the hip in the laboratory lop rabbit: its possible relationship to factors involved in so-called 'congenital dislocation' of the hip. *Clin. Orthop. Relat. Res.* 44: 221-229.

Atrash, H. K., Friede, A., Hogue, C. J. 1987. Abdominal pregnancy in the United States: Frequency and maternal mortality. *Obstet. Gynecol.* 69: 333-337.

Bland-Sutton, J. 1904. Abdominal pregnancy in women, cats, dogs and rabbits. *Lancet* ii 1625-1627.

Bland, K. P., Donovan, B. T. 1965. Experimental ectopic implantation of eggs and early embryos in guinea-pigs. *J. Reprod. Fertil.* 10:189-196.

Bishop, C. R. 2002. Reproductive medicine of rabbits and rodents. *Veterinary Clinics North America: Exotic Animal Practice* 5:507-535.

Buckley, P. and Caine, A. 1979. A high incidence of abdominal pregnancy in the Djungarian hamster (Phodopus sungorus). *J. Rep. and Fert.* 56: 679-682.

Bunte, R. M. and Hildebrandt, P. K. 1975. Abdominal mummified fetus in an owl monkey. *J. Am. Vet. Med. Assoc.* 167: 667-668.

Carlton, A. E., Moore, G. D., Pauerstein, C. 1991. Ectopic pregnancy and tubal refractoriness to implantation in animals. *Arch. Biol. Med. Exp.* 24: 411-416.

Choi, H. K., Atkinson, K., Karlson, E. W., Willet, W., Curham, G. 2004. Purine-rich foods, dairy and protein intake, and the risk of gout in men. *New Engl. J. Med.* 350:1093-1103.

Crownover, R. W., Yeargan, G. S. Jr. 1976. Extra-uterine pregnancy in a spayed cat. *Vet. Med. Small Anim. Clin.* 71(12):1698-1699.

CDC-Centers for Disease Control and Prevention. Ectopic Pregnancy Surveillance, United States, 1970-1985. In: CDC Surveillance Summaries. *Morb. Mort. Wkly. Rep.* 1988; 37(no. SS-5):9SS-18SS.

CDC-Centers for Disease Control and Prevention Ectopic Pregnancy in the United States of America 1978-1989. In: CDC Surveillance Summaries. *Morb. Mortal. Wkly. Rep.* 1992;41:591-594.

CDC-Centers for Disease Control and Prevention. Ectopic Pregnancy–United States, 1990-1992. *MMWR Morb. Mortal. Wkly. Rep.* 1995;44:46-8.

Complications of Pregnancy Part 1. [Internet]. 2007. *Early pregnancy.* Vol. 9 no 6. [Cited 21 September 2012]. Available from: www. ebmedicine.net.

Cosman, M. P., Jones, L. G. 2008. *Handbook to life in the Medieval World.* Infobase Publishing. pp. 2008;528-529.

Coste, J., Bouyer, J., Germain, E., Ughetto, S., Pouly, J. L., Job-Spira, N. 2000. Recent declining trend in ectopic pregnancy in France: evidence of two clinic epidemiologic entities. *Fertil. Steril.* 74: 881-886.

Coste, J., Bouyer, J., Ughetto, S., Gerbaud, L., Fernandez, H., Pouly, J. L., Job-Spira, N. 2004. Ectopic pregnancy is again on the increase. Recent trends in the incidence of ectopic pregnancies in France (1992-2002). *Hum. Rep.* 19 (9): 2014-2017.

Corpa, J. M. 2006. Review: Ectopic pregnancy in animals and humans. *J. Reprod.* 131: 631-640.

Creanga, A. A., Shapiro-Mendoza, C. K., Bish, C. L., Zane, S., Berg, C. J., Callaghan, W. M. 2011. Trends in Ectopic Pregnancy Mortality in the United States 1980-2007. *Obstet. Gynecol.*, 117(4):837-843.

David, R. 2004. Rationality versus irrationality in Egyptian medicine in the pharaonic and Graeco-Roman periods. *Stud. Anc. Med.* 27:133-151.

David, R. 2008. The art of healing in ancient Egypt: a scientific reappraisal. *Lancet* 22; 372 (9652):1802-1803.

Dickie, E. 2011. Dystocia in a rabbit (*Oryctolagus cuniculus*). *Can. Vet. J.* 52 (1) 80-83.

Eales, N. B. 1932. Abdominal pregnancy in animals, with an account of a case of multiple ectopic gestation in a rabbit. *J. Anat.* 67:108-117.

Eddey, F. D. 2012. Ectopic Pregnancy in an Apparently Healthy Bitch. *J. Am. Anim. Hosp. Assoc.* 48:194-197.

Eshar, D., Mayer, J. 2008. An unusual abdominal mass in a rabbit. *Lab. Anim.* (NY); 37:109-111.

Fawcett, D. W., Wislocki, G. B., Waldo, C. M. 1947. The development of mouse ova in the anterior chamber of the eye and in the abdominal cavity. *Am. J. Anat.* 81(3):413-443.

Flatt, R. E., Weisbroth, S. H., Kraus, A. L. 1974. Metabolic, Traumatic, Mycotic, and Miscellaneous Diseases of Rabbits. In: Weisbroth, S. H., Flatt, R. E., Kraus, A. L., Editors. *The Biology of the_Laboratory Rabbit.* New York, Academic Press, pp. 435-451.

Flecknell, P. A. 2000. *Manual of rabbit medicine and surgery,* Gloucester (UK) British Small Animal Veterinary Association. pp. 248-255.

Foote, R. H. 2002. The history of artificial insemination: Selected notes and notables. *J. Anim. Sci.* 80(E. Suppl.):E22-E32.

Gosden, R. G., Russell, J. A. 1981. Spontaneous abdominal implantation in the rat with development to full term. *Lab. Anim.* 15:379.

Hannon, C. A. 1981. Mummified fetuses in a cat. *Modern Vet. Pract.* 62:133-134.

Harcourt-Brown, F. M. 2002. *Textbook of rabbit medicine.* Oxford (UK). Butterworth Heinemamm. pp. 333-351.

Harper, P. A., Ensley, P. K. 1982. Mummified fetus associated with uterine rupture in a New Zealand white rabbit (Oryctolagus cuniculus). *Lab. Anim. Sci.* 32:518-519.

Hasan, I., Zulkifle, M., Ansari, A. H., Sherwani, A. M. K., Shakir, M. 2011. History of Ancient Egyptian Obstetrics and Gynecology: A Review. *J. Microbiol. Biotech. Res.* 1(1): 35-39.

Hong, C. C., Armstrong, M. L. 1978. Ectopic pregnancy in 2 guinea-pigs. *Lab. Anim.* 12: 243-244.

Hreshchyshyn, M. M., Hreshchyshyn, L. O. 1964. Experimentally induced abdominal pregnancy in mice. *Am. J. Obstet. Gynecol.* 89:829-830.

Kamel, R. M. 2013. Assisted Reproductive Technology after the Birth of Louise Brown. *J. Reprod. Infert.* 14(3):96-109.

Kaygusuz, E., Cetiner, H., Yavuz, H., Cesur, S., Yozgatligil, C., Ayas, S. 2014. Immunohistochemical Expressions of Receptors for Luteinizing Hormone/Human Chorionic Gonadotropic Hormone and FOR Sex Steroid Hormones in Pregnant Fallopian Tubes. *Gen. Endocrinol.* 181-194. [Cited 10 August 2014] Available from: http://89.45.199.148/2014/numarul2/fulltext/181-194%20Gen%20Endo%20-%20E.%20Kaygusuz.pdf.

Kobayashi, F., Sagawa, N., Konishi, I. 1996. Spontaneous conception and intrauterine pregnancy in asymptomatic missed abortion of ectopic pregnancy in the previous cycle. *Hum. Reprod.* 11:1347-1349.

Kobayashi, A., Behringer, R. R. 2003. Developmental genetics of the female reproductive tract in mammals. *Nat. Rev. Genet.* 4(12):969-980.

Krugner-Higby, L., Luck, M., Hartley, D., Crispen, H. M., Lubach, G. R., Coe, C. L. 2009. High-risk pregnancy in rhesus monkeys (*Macaca mulatta*): a case of ectopic, abdominal pregnancy with birth of a live, term infant, and a case of gestational diabetes complicated by pre- eclampsia. *J. Med. Primatol.* 38(4):252.

Kuntz, A. A. 1922. A case of abdominal pregnancy with retention of dead fetuses in the rabbit. *Anat. Rec.* 23:237-239.

Lapin, B. A., Yakovleva, L. A. 1963. *Comparative Pathology in Monkeys.* Springfield, Ill, Charles C. Thomas, pp. 216-219.

Lee, R. K. K., Lin, S. P., Tsai, Y. J., Lin, M. H., Hwa, Y. M. 2000. Embryonic dormancy phenomenon in obstructed healthy mouse fallopian tubes. *J. Assist. Reprod. Genet.* 17:540-545.

Levasseur, M. C. 1983. Putative causes of the frequency of extra-uterine pregnancy in women and its rarity in domestic mammals. *Contracep. Fertil. Sexual.* (Paris) 11:1207-1213.

Lim, H. J. and Wang, H. 2010. Uterine disorders and pregnancy complications: insights from mouse models. *J. Clin. Invest.* 120(4):1004-1015. doi:10.1172/JCI41210.

Lin, T. K., Lee, R. K. K., Lin, S. P., Chen, S. Y., Tsai, Y. J., Su, T. H. 2001. Growth retardation of rabbit embryosin ligated oviducts and the toxic effects of rabbit tubal fluid on mouse embryo development *in vitro*. *J. Assist. Reprod. Genet.* 18 (7): 400-405.

Maertens, L., Lebas, F., Szendrö, Zs. 2006. Rabbit Milk: A Review of Quantity, Quality and Non- dietary Affecting Factors. *World Rabb. Sci.* 14:205-230.

McClure, H. M. and Chang, J. 1975. Ectopic pregnancy in a squirrel monkey. *J. Am. Vet. Med. Assoc.* 167:654-655.

Mc Keating, F. J. 1979. Ectopic pregnancy in a cat. *Vet. Rec.* 104:240-241.

Merskey, H., Merskey, S. J. 1993. Hysteria or "suffocation of the mother". *CMAJ*. 148(3):399-405.

Mitchell, K. W. 1989. Ectopic pregnancy in a ewe. *Vet. Rec.* 124:498-452.

Newbatt, E., Beckles, Z., Ullman, R., Lumsden, M. A. 2012. Guideline Development Group. Ectopic pregnancy and miscarriage: summary of NICE guidance. *BMJ*, 345:e8136. doi:10.1136/bmj.e8136.

Nour, F. O. M. *Ectopic pregnancy Incidence, Morbidity and Mortality. 2010.* [Cited 10 August 2014] Available from: http://www.gfmer.ch/Endo/Fellows_11/Pdf/Ectopic_pregnancy.pdf.

Odewale, M. A. and Afolabi, M. O. 2008. Heterotopic pregnancy: a clinical case report from rural Nigeria. *Rur. and Remot. Health* 8:979. [Cited 22 September 2012]. Available from: http://rrh.org.au.

Ohlman, D. 2010. *The Natural Order*. [Cited 15 October 2010] Available from: http://wonderofcreation.org/2010/10/15/the-natural-order/

Owensby, T., Jackson, K., Scharf, B. 2001. Failure to deliver in a rabbit with intra-abdominal masses. *Lab. Anim.* 30:23-25.

Petraglia, F., Bettini, M. 2010. Human reproduction in art: from myths to history. *Rep. Sci.* 17(8):711-717.

Pisarska, M. D., Carson, S. A., Buster, J. E. 1998. Ectopic pregnancy. *Lancet* 351:1115-1120.

Polysciences Inc. [Cited 10 August 2014] Available from: http://www.polysciences.com/Catalog/Department/Product/98/categoryid--28/productid. 326/

Pulkkinen, M. O. 1995. Oviductal function is critical for very early human life. *Annals of Med.* 2:7 307-310.

Rabinerson, D. D., Pollak-Rabinerson, N. N., Glezerman, M. M. 2008. Superfecundation and superfetation - the forgotten entities. *Harefuah* 147 (2):155-158,181. [Article in Hebrew].

Rajkhowa, M., Rutherford, A. J., Sharma, V., Glass, M. R., Balen, A. H., Cuckle, H. S. 2000. Trends in the incidence of ectopic pregnancy in England and Wales from 1966 to 1996. *Brit. J. Obst. and Gynaecol.* 107: 369-374.

Rana, P., Kazmi, I., Singh, R., Afzal, M., Al-Abbasi, F. A., Aseeri, A., Singh, R., Khan, R., Anwar, F. 2013. Ectopic pregnancy: a review. *Arch. Gynecol. Obstet.* 288:745-757.

Rosset, E., Galet, C., Buff, S. 2011. A case report of an ectopic fetus in a cat. *J. Fel. Med. and Surg.* 13(8): 610-613.

Saifudeen, Z., Liu, J., Dipp, S., Yao, X., Li, Y., et al. 2012. A p53-Pax2 pathway in kidney development: Implications for nephrogenesis. *PLoS ONE* 7(9): e44869. doi: 10.1371// journal.pone.0044869.

Sasidharan, K., Dutta, S., Narang, A. Validity of New Ballard Score until 7th day of postnatal life in moderately preterm neonates. *Arch. Dis. Child. Fet. Neonat.* 2009; 94(1):F39-44. doi: 10.1136/adc.2007.122564.

Schlabritz-Loutsevitch, N. E., Hubbard, G. B., Frost, P. A., Cummins, L. B., Dick, E. J., Jr, Nathanielsz, P. W., McDonald, T. J. 2004. Abdominal pregnancy in a baboon: a first case report. *J. Med. Primatol.* 33:55-59.

Segura-Gil, P., Peris-Palau, B., Martínez-Martínez, J., Ortega-Porcel, J., Corpa-Arenas, J. M. 2004. Abdominal pregnancies in farm rabbits. *Theriogenol.* 62:642-651.

Shafi, S. M., Malla, M. A., Salaam, P. A., Kirmani, O. S. 2009. Abdominal pregnancy as a cause of hemoperitoneum. *J. Emerg. Trauma Shock.* 2(3): 196-198.

Shao, R. 2010. Understanding the mechanisms of human tubal ectopic pregnancies: new evidence from knockout mouse models. *Hum. Reprod.* 25:584-587.

Shaw, J. L., Dey, S. K., Critchley, H. O., Horne, A. W. 2010. Current knowledge of the aetiology of human tubal ectopic pregnancy. *Hum. Reprod. Update.* 16:432-444.

Simms, I., Rogers, P. A., Nicoll, A. 1997. The influence of demographic change and cumulative risk of pelvic inflammatory disease on the incidence of ectopic pregnancy. *Epidemiol. Infect.* 119(1):49-52.

Slavotinek, A., Biesecker, L. G. 2003. Genetic modifiers in human development and malformation syndromes, including chaperone proteins. *Hum. Mol. Genetics* 12, Review Issue 1 R45-R50. DOI: 10.1093/hmg/ddg 099.

Tay, J. I., Moore, J., Walker, J. J. 2000. Ectopic pregnancy. *West. J. Med.* 2000; 173(2):131-134.

Tena-Betancourt, E., Tena-Betancourt, C. A., Zúniga-Muñoz, A. M., Hernández-Godínez, B., Ibáñez-Contreras, A., Graullera-Rivera, V. 2014. Multiple extrauterine pregnancy with early and near full-term mummified fetuses in a New Zealand White Rabbit (*Oryctolagus cuniculus*). *J. Am. Ass. Lab. Anim. Sci.* 53(2):204-207.

Tena-Betancourt, E., Hernández-Godínez, B., Ibañez-Contreras, A., Reyes-Pantoja, S., Graullera-Rivera, V., Pérez-González, R. 2012. Superfetación en una coneja Nueva Zelanda Blanca (*Oryctolagus cuniculus*) concomitante a evento de distocia materna: Reporte Preliminar. *Abstracts presented at the X Encuentro Nacional de Cunicultura*, Oaxaca, Mexico, 1-3 October 2012. [CD-ROM]. Memorias, X Encuentro Nacional de Cunicultura 1:56.

Tena, E., García-Formentí, E., Aldúcin, R., Hernández, R., Tena, C. 1991. Multiple ectopic pregnancy in a New Zealand white rabbit (*Oryctolagus cuniculus*). *Abstracts of scientific papers: AALAS/ ICLAS joint meeting*, Buffalo, New York, 20-24 October 1991. Cordova (TN): American Association for Laboratory Animal Science.

Tena-Betancourt, E., Hernández-Godínez, B., Ibáñez-Contreras, A., Reyes--Pantoja, S., Zúñiga-Muñoz, A.M.,Graullera-Rivera,V.2013. Posible superfetación en una coneja raza N.Z.B. (Oryctolagus cuniculus) concomitante a retraso del desarrollo intrauterino (RDIU). Spei Domus 9 (19):49-56.

Wang, H., Guo, Y., Wang, D., Kingsley, P. J., Marnett, L. J., Das, S. K., DuBois, R. N., Dey, S. K. 2004. Aberrant cannabinoid signaling impairs oviductal transport of embryos. *Nat. Med.* 10(10):1074-1080.

Van Den Eeden, S. K., Shan, J., Bruce, C., Glasser, M. 2005. Ectopic pregnancy rate and treatment utilization in a large managed care organization. *Obst. and Gynecol.* 105:1052-1057.

Zotte Dalle and Szendro, Z. 2011. The role of rabbit meat as functional food. *Meat Sci.* 88(3):319-331. doi: 10.1016/j.meatsci.2011.02.017. Epub. 2011 Feb. 24.

About the Authors

Eduardo Tena-Betancourt, DVM, MSc. Coordinator of Animal Facility Services and Experimental Surgery, Mexican Faculty of Medicine, La Salle University Mexico, México D.F., C.P. 14000. Professor, Department of Ethology, Wildlife and Laboratory Animals, Faculty of Veterinary Medicine and Zootechnics, Ciudad Universitaria, Coyoacán, México D.F. C.P. 04510. E-mail: eduardo.tena@ulsa.mx.

Braulio Hernández-Godínez. Phys. Antropologist: Researcher, BIOINVERT®. Biología Integral para Vertebrados: Unidad de Experimentación Animal, Edo. México, México. E-mail: rhpithecus@ yahoo.com.mx.

Alejandra Ibáñez-Contreras, DVM, MSc: Researcher, BIOINVERT®. Biología Integral para Vertebrados: Unidad de Experimentación Animal, Edo. México, México. E-mail: ibanez.alejandra@hotmail.com.

Verónica Graullera-Rivera, DVM. Staff Veterinarian, Department of Pathology, I.N.C. "Ignacio Chávez", México D.F., C.P. 14050. E-mail: grauvero@yahoo.com.mx.

Daniel Muñoz-Jiménez, M.D. Research Assistant, Mexican Faculty of Medicine, La Salle University Mexico, México D.F., C.P. 14000. E-mail: daniel@emjou.com.

Index

A

B

C

D

E

F

G

H

M

N

O

P

Q

R

S

T

U